Intimate
adventures
of an
office
girl

Intimate
adventures
of an
office
girl

**An ordinary girl,
an extraordinary
sex life...**

SIENNA LEWIS

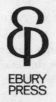

EBURY
PRESS

1 3 5 7 9 10 8 6 4 2

First published in 2009 by Ebury Press, an imprint of Ebury
Publishing
A Random House Group company

Copyright © Sienna Lewis 2009

Sienna Lewis has asserted her right to be identified as the
author of this Work in accordance with the Copyright, Designs
and Patents Act 1988

The Random House Group Limited Reg. No. 954009

Addresses for companies within the Random House Group can be
found at www.randomhouse.co.uk

A CIP catalogue record for this book is available from
the British Library

The Random House Group Limited supports The Forest Stewardship
Council (FSC), the leading international forest certification
organisation. All our titles that are printed on Greenpeace approved
FSC certified paper carry the FSC logo. Our paper procurement
policy can be found at www.rbooks.co.uk/environment

Printed in the UK by CPI Cox & Wyman, Reading, RG1 8EX

ISBN 9780091928827

To buy books by your favourite authors and register for offers visit
www.rbooks.co.uk

Disclaimer

This book is a work of non-fiction based on the life, experiences and recollections of the author. The names of people, places, dates, sequences or the detail of events have been changed to protect the privacy of others.

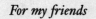

For my friends

Contents

Preface   1

1 Ladies' Choice   5

2 Horizontal Communication 27

3 The Soulless Soulmate 52

4 The Game 86

5 Absinthe for Breakfast 114

6 Diving for Pearls 143

7 Kensington Nights 158

8 Be My Baby 186

9 Office Romance 219

10 Doctors and Nurses 250

11 New Babies, Old Feelings 268

12 Truth or Dare 289

Epilogue 302

Acknowledgements 305

Preface

The office is quiet. No post, no phone calls, no computer crashes, no reason to complain about the cleaner, and our accountant is not due in for another two weeks or so. Nothing for me to do – I might as well kick my feet up on my desk and file my nails before lunchtime. Yet here I am typing away at my top speed of 55–60 wpm, a slow smile spreading on my face, cheeks flushed with the memory of the night before.

My boss interrupts what he's doing (probably reading and replying to all his junk mail: 'Would U l1ke a Biga Pen15?') and looks over at me with a puzzled expression:

'Are you writing a book?'

'Maybe,' I reply, trying to remain cool. Fortunately I've chosen the desk where nobody can see my computer screen. I quickly open my Outlook, just in case (no new messages). He goes back to what he was doing (watching people fly off mountains on YouTube) and ignores me. I don't think he believed me.

After all, what could I possibly be doing that was worth writing about? Filing? Redecorating my flat? Juggling multiple lovers, an addiction to internet dating, a proposal, and an unrequited passion? Well, I suppose my boss wouldn't have guessed that about me; I'm a little surprised about it myself, but then again, I always thought I'd grow up to be a girl who enjoys sex.

At the age of eleven, I discovered my parents' 1970s sex-book collection neatly arranged in alphabetical order on the shelves below Freud, Kant and Tolstoy. I'd snatch one or more of them on my way to the bathroom and lock myself in for extensive reading sessions, poring over the pages and the diagrams.

I drew a school friend into my confidence and one Saturday afternoon when she came round to see me I broke out my latest discovery in adult-interest non-fiction. We were sitting on my bed and flicking through the pages when we came to a photograph of a woman sitting across a man, both of them naked. 'That's how my mum was sitting on her boyfriend,' she confessed. 'I saw them through the keyhole one afternoon.'

Woman on top? Afternoon sex? Could it get any more debauched? And my friend had actually seen this! I felt myself getting excited. 'When I look at these images,' she admitted, 'I get a funny tingling down below.' I admired her confidence in confessing this, as I felt the same but didn't dare mention it.

At school, my friends and I had begun swapping trashy romance novelettes with sentimental titles, soft-focus covers and red-hot content. They were full of dashing, arrogant architects 'roughly taking' the construction magnate's aloof and elegant daughter in dilapidated buildings, shy nannies and wealthy landowners getting caught in the rain without a horse, and other such nonsense.

Of course, the first kiss usually led to marriage and penetration invariably to an earth-shattering orgasm, which wasn't enough detail for us, so we tried to re-create this world of adult delights in our own words. We produced our own trashy novels, filling the pages with our own fantasies supplemented by my raids on my parents' sex manuals. We were less bothered with the marriage and white frocks, and more concerned with allowing our heroines dramatic and semi-consensual sex lives. I might have been behind physically – I was annoyingly flat and bare in all the important places, envying my friends' smattering of pubes and blooming breasts when they were revealed in the showers – but my stories were popular!

I discovered masturbation by reading about it in my parents' books. Knowing the ins and outs in theory was one thing, getting myself off in reality quite another. I tried rubbing against a pillow, a pen and even flicking a feather across my clit, all with rather disappointing results.

'How do you manage to touch yourself?' I asked another friend, Judy, disgusted by the thought of putting my bare hand 'there'. She told me she used rubber gloves, and gave me a pair she'd nicked from her parents' medicine cupboard. Immediately, things improved and I felt more comfortable exploring myself. Now, of course, I chuckle at the thought. The places my once-innocent hands have been since then!

Judy and I created a fantasy world of macho motorcycling boyfriends, rough sex, betrayal and getting lost by our men in poker games, to be shared by the rest of the gang. Her imaginary boyfriend was loosely based on Tom Cruise in *Top Gun*, mine looked like a guy I'd once seen in a black-and-white afternoon TV movie. That's until I discovered Patrick Swayze and *Dirty Dancing*.

Unable to choose between the fictional, sexy and predatory Patrick and my reliable, sensitive boyfriend Don (represented by an old pillow), I embarked on an unconventional affair with both of them. Even at the age of thirteen, I had to have my cake and eat it.

Fast forward fifteen years and I'm living the life I used to daydream about. After a bad break-up I gave up on monogamy and opened my heart, mind and legs to men who may not tick all the boxes but certainly tickle my fancy, and while I don't live in a permanent state of threesome happiness, my flatmate likes to joke that I'd benefit from installing a revolving door on my bedroom.

It's been one hell of a ride, so I began keeping notes so I wouldn't get confused – and about a year and a half ago I started an online blog charting my sexual successes and failures in London's dating jungle. I wanted to record honestly every single sexual adventure I had, the good, the bad and the ugly, the highs and the lows. This is it.

1

Ladies' Choice

Monday 15th August

OK. Here goes.

My name is Sienna.

I've got a pretty ordinary job in advertising that means I work in a pretty ordinary office in London from nine to five-thirty. I rent a flat without a living room in a scruffy part of East London which is slowly becoming 'trendy' with a flatmate who thinks the kitchen cleans itself. I don't want to give too much away about my everyday life so I can be as honest as possible in this blog, but I could be the receptionist in your building, the person bidding against you on an account, or the girl next to you on the bus reading her stars in *Metro*. I could be your best friend, or your ex. The girl on the dating site you haven't got round to clicking on yet. I'm twenty-seven with shoulder-length blonde curly hair, and I'm tall but not skinny; I like to drink cocktails in the West End and go dancing with my friends and while I like the regular hours of my job, I'd also like to do some more freelance writing on the side. I was born in a small town outside of London and brought up in continental Europe by liberal, financially challenged parents who thankfully divorced when I was a teenager. At eighteen I moved to London for love and university. The love part didn't work out, but uni furnished me with a 2:1 in something creative, which I am now trying to use in my career. I want to get married and have babies at some point, too, but that means I'll have to find the right guy first. Oh, and I spent this weekend with two different men – and the one before that – but I'm not cheating on either of them. More about them tomorrow, but I should probably explain my dating philosophy first.

A few months ago I had a disastrous break up with a boyfriend I'll call Pinocchio, whom I'd practically lived with for the best part of nine months before he turned out to be, well, a little wooden man who told lies. I was left to carry my heart home in a carrier bag and now I'm a little sceptical about the conventional way of finding Mr Right. You see, I still believe in husbands. I believe in lovers. One's exclusive, the others are not. I just don't believe in boyfriends any more – what are they supposed to be?

Someone you're idiotically faithful to without the commitment of marriage? A guy who wastes your time while a dozen other dreamboats sail past you in the night? Whoever said that an exclusive relationship starts the minute you jump into bed with someone? When did we stop assuming that it does?

At some point I just stopped believing that there is any kind of convention for modern relationships at all. Men are no longer producing rings and vows of eternal troth the minute they want to get into your knickers, preferring instead the route of least resistance (and expense) that comes from pulling someone when she's drunk. Of course, keeping her number is optional.

Further down the line, provided he did keep her number and she cares about seeing him again, the woman might want to initiate 'the conversation' – are we an item, and if yes, what does this involve?

Men don't usually like this conversation, which is great as long as you are also not sure if you'd like to see him exclusively. So you don't. After all it takes a while to get to know someone, and it would be a shame to pass up on all those other opportunities that tend to present themselves if you like to go out, know how to use the internet and are curious about meeting new people.

Who said we have to stop trying before we've 'bought'?

Rather than waiting to sleep with someone until we're married, which is no longer expected of anyone outside religious communities, we should take advantage of being able to sleep with as many people as we like before we decide to commit to just one.

You could call what I'm doing 'multiple dating' or 'spreading your bets'.

I can't claim to have invented the notion. My friend Canada Boy told me about it first.

I met him at a friend's work party after returning from a depressing business trip, and although he was into my friend at first I liked him straight away. We began to sort of see each other – meeting for drinks, flirting, kissing – but I always held back, wary of getting involved with someone too soon after my split with Pinocchio. Somehow we mixed a growing friendship undercut with a kind of erotic tension with long boozing sessions in bars where he'd tell me how 'hot' I made him, and would squeeze my thigh under the table so I could feel his excitement, and he'd breathlessly run through a list of all the nooks and crannies in his office where we could fuck, or how he was going to pull me under the pool table right now and lick my pussy wet. At some stage these fantasies drifted off into the ridiculous, but there was never any aggression from him when I left alone – he knew I was already seeing someone else, and I suspected he was involved with someone, too. I knew he was still obsessing over his ex, and he understood that I'd had my heart broken and liked him too much to risk ruining our friendship.

Besides, I seemed to be shying away from real intimacy. I'd started to see a really nice guy after my break-up, but after three months of dating and snogging, I could tell he was, not surprisingly, getting bored. I thought I was doing it all right – you know, getting to know him, making sure I was in Luuurve with a capital L before tumbling into bed – but the Nice Guy got bored and stopped calling. In a funny way I was relieved because I could tell things weren't 100 per cent right between us and it was just too early for me to settle into another relationship.

Canada Boy offered me a way to let go of my hang ups, along with a few of my expectations. One evening he and I crossed the line from friends with flirting privileges to soulmates, and I confessed to him that, after my ex, I didn't see the point of fully committing myself to anyone unless they'd invested three months' salary in a piece of carbon – isn't sexual fidelity a marriage promise? Canada Boy just smiled and shrugged and said, 'What you're talking about sounds a bit like polyamory. You are free to have several lovers at the same time who know about each other, rather than be unhappy and dishonest with just the one. I'd rather have two girlfriends who fancied each other than try to commit to one – that would be pretty unrealistic long-term.'

'Isn't that cheating?' I said. 'I don't want to screw anyone over, just don't want to get hurt myself.'

'It's not cheating if you're up front about it and tell them what's going on. It's their choice to be involved.'

I began to wonder whether I really could have more than one lover if I were totally honest about it. I didn't plan to be a bitch and rub their noses in it, but they'd be free to come and go as they liked, so there would be none of the pressure of a committed relationship.

After all, every girl I know has more than one good girlfriend, and no one has a problem with us spending quality time with each of those friends in turn. If you're talking about men and women and you throw sex into the equation, why does that automatically have to mean we get all possessive and monogamous? I mean, why bother to stick to one guy if you don't know if he's The One?

Relying on one man to give me everything – to love me, phone me, listen to me bitch about work, rub my feet, whisk me away to a hotel, to be everything I wanted in bed – and me giving him all my time and affection and spending hours thinking up little things to make him happy – that wasn't working. I needed some time out of the battle till I felt better about myself and could trust someone again.

Canada Boy was right. Instead of having one relationship after another with them all ending with me in therapy and the boyfriend tucked up with another woman, why not have all my relationships develop at the same time?

I mean, just think about the advantages:

+ No more waiting by the phone. If he doesn't call,
  who cares? One of the others will.
+ If he's not free to see me, I don't have to nag him or
  worry that he's with someone else because I'll be with
  someone else too.
+ No messing around wondering whether you can ask
  if you're seeing each other 'exclusively' or if that
  makes you sound like a marriage-obsessed stalker
  who wants to talk about matching place cards at the
  wedding after one date.

- No putting your eggs in one basket, knowing there's a whole world of other baskets (and basketcases) out there waiting.
- No playing games and withholding sex in order to see if someone's 'serious'. Why shouldn't I sleep with whoever I want to, and satisfy my own libido? I'm not a nun, and holding back from Nice Guy had left me horny. If I am truly free, I can have all the sex I want without emotional complications.

I'm not on some revenge trip against mankind. I like men after all – too much! – and they're not my enemies. A little bit of discretion was needed, I thought, and a lot of organisation. Plus of course they get plenty out of it too – if I'm not obsessed with whether I can share a bed with them until we're ninety and have seven great grandchildren or if they have annoying habits like leaving their pants sunny-side up all over the floor, then I'm going to be a whole lot more tolerant of any imperfections. We'll have a good time, and if either of us is having a bad day the other one doesn't have to deal with it. If either of us wants more we'll have to come out with it and ask – no more mind reading and getting it wrong. It sounds simple enough, right?

My best friend, Samantha, recommended a dating site which had helped her up her tally from seventy-five to ninety-eight, so I fired up my computer, loaded up a profile and waited to see what happened.

Tuesday 16th August

So the two guys I mentioned earlier I'll call the Pilot and Porsche Boy – the nicknames are a bit of a giveaway. They don't know about each other *precisely*, but if I choose to spend

Saturday with the boy who's in love with his sports car and Sunday with my pilot, there's no problem. It feels naughty and weird to be so popular but I'm only following my own code. Here's a bit of background on them.

I met the Pilot at an airport, of course. I was on my way back from a family funeral, carrying a wok my mum had thoughtfully bought for me, and he was on his way back from visiting an ex-girlfriend. We'd both passed through check-in and passport control and were milling around waiting for our flight. I didn't know we'd be sharing a plane later, just clocked this incredibly handsome blond guy sipping a coffee, who was smiling at me. I smiled back and retreated into the newsagents.

I don't know why I had a hunch that he'd follow me into the shop, but I picked up a scuba-diving magazine instead of *Glamour* or *Cosmo* so he didn't think I was superficial or obsessed with sex or the size of my hips, and sure enough he came up to me and asked me something about diving. It turned out that he'd just finished his Open Water qualification in Egypt, a place I wanted to go to, and we were off.

When our flight was called I had to struggle through security with my unwieldy wok, only to find him on the other side. It felt like we were old friends. I've rarely felt so excited about meeting someone and just couldn't stop looking at his clear green eyes, as he told me about spending his weekends flying his little two-seater plane over Berkshire. He explained that he wants to be a commercial pilot eventually, and it'll take him four years to qualify once he's got the funding.

'And what do you do in the meantime?' I asked, fascinated by him, and when he told me he worked as a security guard, it was the last answer I expected to hear because he seemed a bit too intellectual for that type of job. He told me that his workmates laugh at him for reading broadsheets rather than the *Sunday Sport*.

We talked all the way to London, sitting right at the back of the plane with me by the window, and he filled me in on aerobatics, near misses, deadly crashes and buzzing over to the Isle of Wight for fun. Once he'd worked with a maverick hot air balloon crew, travelling the country holding the rope on those giant balloons used for advertising.

I talked to him about London, which, being a country boy, he didn't know very well. I told him about boat trips on the Thames and he liked the idea – he asked for my phone number at baggage collection, and I didn't hesitate to write it down for him. As I walked off to the tube I felt like breaking into a laugh. It was the first time in a long while that I'd felt such an immediate attraction to someone and found them attracted to me too. I was caught up in the romance of the circumstances – a handsome pilot approaching me in a foreign airport, maybe ready to fly me away for the weekend!

We went swimming in the ponds at Hampstead Heath on our first date, and ended up, a few hours later, having our first kiss under the Eros statue in Piccadilly. The next weekend he took me up in his plane, which was amazing and terrifying. He even let me take the controls for a while and learn how to coordinate my hands and feet to keep the plane in the air. We flew over the Henley Regatta, peering down on the marquees and crowds by the ribbon of the Thames.

When we were back on the ground he drove me to his cottage, and we got drunk on vintage champagne, then I suggested a walk in the meadow that lay on the other side of the garden. I knew what I wanted – a tumble in the long grass – but I wasn't sure about him. He seemed a little uptight, not the type to abandon himself when the mood took him – he'd prefer candlelight in a bedroom to bright sunshine and a light breeze on his bum. I don't think the possibility of an *al fresco* fuck had occurred to him before I pulled him down on top of me and kissed him.

We were hidden by the grass, but as he slipped down and pulled up my skirt to slowly work his tongue under my knicker elastic, I couldn't help wondering if any of the pilots taking off from the airfield nearby were getting an eyeful. His tongue burrowed and flicked – him taking his time, me lazy with the champagne – then he pulled me up and I sat on his lap facing him, my legs wrapped round him and my long skirt rucked up. I undid his jeans and thought for a split second I wasn't going to be wet enough to let him slip into me – he was bigger than I'd expected – but I was more turned on than I'd thought. He fucked me silently, with long, careful strokes, pushing me gently onto my back against the crushed grass. He came and I came a few seconds later, and we sprawled together, still dressed, grass seeds in my hair and insects crawling up my legs, my head on his chest. 'That was nice,' I told him with a grin. He smiled back.

After a while we got up and walked hand in hand back to his cottage and after dinner he lured me up to his bedroom and put an Enya CD on, which almost ruined everything. Seriously, Enya? My evil first boyfriend used to play that; hadn't the Pilot updated his shag tunes in the last decade? Ah well – almost a perfect summer romance in the making, and I wasn't going to let his taste in music rob me of his slow, delicious fucking. Since then I've tried to see him whenever his work shifts allow, and he's free.

Porsche Boy was an acquisition from my internet-dating spree. To be honest, just now I'm not sure what attracted me to him, but superficially he seems to tick all the boxes: single, tall, blond with blue eyes, good job in a multinational corporation, his own flat, an easy manner and a good sense of humour. I suppose he seemed sociable and like he wasn't going to mess around if he wanted to be serious. Just from chatting to him I've learned that most of his friends are married and settling down to have kids and live well-adjusted adult lives in the nicer parts of South London.

We went on a few interesting dinner dates a couple of months ago, then cinema outings, and conversation flowed easily. When we ran out of things to say we snogged endlessly instead of watching the films. I'd try and insist on at least buying the popcorn when he tried to pay for everything – just because his parents own a yacht, didn't mean I wanted him to feel like a meal ticket. I see him about once a week now, sometimes more.

There are flies hovering over the ointment, though. For a start, his 'stalker' ex from the same dating site. I tend to take the side of any 'stalker' whose requests sound reasonable, especially when all they want is closure. I don't think it's possible for someone to let go unless they have a real explanation, and I don't think it's too much for her to ask Porsche Boy for a coffee. After all, they'd shared a few orgasms. Does a quick trip to Starbucks constitute undue encouragement? But he just ignored the text messages from her, hoping she'd get the message.

The other thing is his little habit of calling me 'young lady' like he's my disciplinarian uncle, or he's forgotten my name. Is two years really that much of an age gap, or will he pack it in if I start calling him 'young man' or 'old fart'?

Last Saturday he offered to pick me up from my flat in the evening and drive me to a house party out in the sticks. We arranged a time, but I'd just stepped off the bus after a trip across the city to see a friend when I spotted the gleaming Porsche outside my front door, *fifteen minutes early*. What? I count ten minutes late as 'on time' and can think of a million things to do in the two minutes before I leave the house, and I was desperate to get in my front door, wash my hair and slap a little make-up on before I saw him. No chance. My neighbourhood isn't the kind of area where brand new sports cars with personalised number plates sprout on every street corner. I took three steps past the bus stop and my phone rang – Porsche Boy, sitting in his car outside my house, letting me know he was sitting in his car outside my house.

So I felt hassled, scooting round my flat stuffing things into bags and grabbing a few bits and bobs from the fridge; I had a brain full of things I had to do, and I'd wanted to be excited to see him, and enjoy how excited *he* was about his 'fast car'. I don't care that much about cars, but it meant a lot to him, even though where I grew up Porsches meant mid-life crises. Apparently getting a flashy car is a perk of Porsche Boy's job, and if he can be bothered to get up early he'll even drive it to work, dodging London traffic. Except that he likes Magic FM. So there we were in his smart car, bombing along the motorway listening to granddad music. After the millionth replay of 'Wonderful World' I tried to change the station but he didn't like it, so I had to sit on my hands.

'I hope you didn't mind me driving fast,' he asked me when we arrived. Fast? I hadn't noticed. Aren't fast cars designed so that you don't notice how fast you're going? Ninety mph is the average speed in the middle lane in Germany where my dad lived, so I hadn't really been aware.

The party was a bit boring. He spent most of his time chatting to friends and refused to dance with me. Another guest at this party turned out to be a good friend's brother who was surprised to see me there in the company of Porsche Boy. 'You know,' he told me in a confidential whisper, 'he's a bit of a ladies' man . . .' I could only smile. After all, doesn't that make me 'a gentlemen's woman'?

We were staying in a hotel that night and I got out the whipped cream and strawberries I'd remembered to snatch from the fridge before he could rev his engine too many times. We broke the bed. I think that made up for Magic FM.

He had to leave early on Sunday to catch a flight so I reported the damage at reception while I was standing next to his very overweight single friend. God knows what they thought, but the receptionist didn't look too surprised. Then I had to get back to London in time to meet the Pilot.

Wednesday 17th August

One thing about my new-found love life is that when you're not just focused on one guy, but falling in and out of bed with several, you really notice the differences between them. When I met Chubby Boy in a pub in Edinburgh last week, I wouldn't have guessed that he gave unbelievable head. Incredible, intense conversation, yes, but when he went down on me later that night I practically pulled his ears off I came so hard. Just the thought of it is making me grin like a maniac.

Another thing about him is that he looks great in clothes, really tall and strong, especially when he picked me up and carried me over to his bed, but once he was stripped down there's just no way of getting over the fact that he is properly fat. I'm not talking a tiny beer belly, but flabby, with back fat, and I know that makes me sound like a bitch but I'm trying to be totally honest here. Before we got a cab back to his flat (my uni friend who I was staying with was thankfully supportive of this little escapade) I'd been fantasising about his weight on me, and how tender and sexy it would be to be folded up in a hug and crushed, but it was more like a recipe for an early heart attack. And when we were screwing with him on top, his arms started to hurt and get tired from his own weight. He took ages to come, too, and had to finish himself off in the end, which is never a turn on for a girl.

The other thing is he wants to be serious, and that's just impossible. He lives hundreds of miles away and he's four years younger than me, for God's sake! If I told him I want to start having kids in a couple of years I bet he'd run a mile. Though I always wanted to marry someone in a kilt . . .

Porsche Boy, who picked me up from the airport in London the next day, noticed how tired I was, but that didn't stop us from having a little 'welcome back' tumble in my bed.

The Pilot hasn't called since Sunday, even though I know he's had time off work . . . If I weren't having so much fun trying out all the boys on offer I'd tell myself to get a grip because otherwise I might be in danger of falling for him, even though he's a penniless security guard. He's the most patient, perfect lover I have ever had. He takes his time, lays me out like a precious buffet and kisses, strokes and licks me all over – I never knew I had so many erogenous zones. He kisses my lips like a girl – no sucking and not much tongue, just soft, sweet butterfly pecks. Oh and then there's his sandy, wild hair, his clear green eyes (which I wish he'd keep open when we're having sex), gorgeous lips, the way he slouches a little because he's so tall and lean.

He's the sort of man I could fall in love with, he's so close to perfect, but then there's a downside or two. To drop the delicacy and get to the nitty-gritty, he has a humungous dick, which you might think is great, but it's not. For a start, ordinary condoms don't fit him. I had to go out and buy a job lot of Durex 56 mm (did you know all the packs have measurements on the back? I didn't till the Pilot explained it) and they're not really long enough, either.

And then I swear there's something about penile hydraulics, but it's hard work getting him fully erect. I get very frustrated if he's spent ages going down on me and I just want him inside me *now* and then I've got to stroke him and lick him till he can, and all the time these little evil thoughts are going through my head like, 'Am I too fat to turn him on? Doesn't he fancy me? Is he thinking about the football?' and we're already on the third CD. Please, if you get into bed with me, be nice and hard and turned on – just the feel of that against the small of my back makes me wet.

Actually, I discovered the real trick to helping him finally come – making him keep his socks on. That's my tip for success. They can't get their rocks off if their feet are cold, I swear. In winter, I sometimes keep my socks on too – same principle!

Also, incidentally, he says I give the 'world's best blow jobs, ever'. Anyway, once he's finally ready he doesn't go on for too long or come straight away, so I get to come again for a second time, which is glorious, but he likes to make a lot of noise and breathe hard in my ears. Somehow I'm guessing his ex got really turned on by that, and it's kinda sexy but it's a bit theatrical for me. I never get much sleep because of all that long-drawn-out cinematic love making, and it's a bit of a disadvantage when some-times a girl just wants, y'know, a quick, filthy bang in the kitchen or a surprise when she bends over in the shower. Porsche Boy is different. He's the same height as the Pilot – any taller and neither of them would fit in my shower – but he's a totally different shape, bulky, in a not-too-muscly way. He's got lovely, fluffy blond fur on his arms and legs but a smooth chest (the Pilot has three chest hairs – I counted them). He has gingery pubes and when his dick is flaccid it looks really tiny nestling in them, but it's average size when it's erect. He uses Durex too, incidentally.

He's a funny one, Porsche Boy. I don't feel very close to him emotionally, and even in bed he can be quite cold. It gets on my nerves that he never really goes for it, just keeps warning me he's going to come, and I've got to stop moving or he *will* come, and I'm just lying there thinking, 'Keep going, go *harder*, go faster!' while I'm pulling him deeper into me, wanting to feel him bang into me so I get something out of it too, but he keeps holding back and it's enormously frustrating.

Then he comes anyway after barely a minute despite his restraint, and I'm thinking, hello? What about me? But then he's hard again almost straight away, which is essential if you were only halfway there the first time.

The other drawback is that he likes sixty-nine, and I've got a few issues with that:

- I once read that women bite down involuntarily when they orgasm, and I can't get that thought out of my head.
- Does he find it boring to go down on a woman without having her sucking on his dick? Hmmm . . .
- The view.
- My brain is so busy concentrating on what my tongue is doing that I can never just switch off and come (and bite his penis off by accident . . .)

Although maybe sixty-nine would be different with the Pilot. I love the feeling of his dick in my mouth . . . On Sunday I got my period after my bed-breaking adventure with Porsche Boy, and I hadn't meant to sleep with the Pilot, but he has this habit of pushing all my buttons at once, and he didn't mind and went down on me just the same and it was the perfect cure for period pains. (To anyone who finds this gross, I'd just like to repeat a quote from my older – and wiser – friend Alexander on the subject: 'If you're going to the theatre you don't have to walk around the whole of the West End.')

For the second time after sleeping with the Pilot I was so happy that I actually cried ... After we'd been cuddling and gazing at each other like lovesick, pink fluffy bunnies for a bit, he got rid of the (literally) bloody condom and started to get dressed. Pretending to myself I was just curious, I decided to ask him in a casual way what was stopping him having a girlfriend. I know my own reasons for staying out of a conventional relationship at the moment, but what were his? He said something about 'time constraints' (he works funny hours) and 'not being very good at keeping in touch'.

Right, this from a man who confesses to maintaining a four-year long-distance relationship – how would that have worked if he hadn't put the time and effort in to phone, travel and write to her? It did explain why he hadn't called me for ages though, and I suppose I wasn't exactly gathering dust on the shelf while he was away.

He had to leave after that, with his uniform bag in hand, and the telephone repair man arrived at the same time so I looked like a desperate housewife in a cheap porno flick – one in, one out! The telephone repair guy took a shine to me and told me about a secret restaurant in Camden where a bottle of Perrier Rosé champagne costs £35. I think I'll bear that in mind for when the Sailor comes to visit. I'll try not to think about what the Pilot said.

Thursday 18th August

Things I still miss about Pinocchio:

- ◆ Reading next to him in bed.
- ◆ Cuddling on the sofa.

- ◆ Brushing his cat.
- ◆ How comfortable I always felt in his flat.
- ◆ The incredible sex.
- ◆ His dick.
- ◆ Stroking his smooth back.
- ◆ His lovely chest and bum.
- ◆ His lips, his eyes.
- ◆ Wearing his bathrobe.
- ◆ Laughing together. So much laughing.
- ◆ Feeling really close to him and loved.
- ◆ Eating together.
- ◆ My head on his chest.
- ◆ 'Our favourite drink.'
- ◆ Waking up together.

How can I still feel like this? The last time I saw him (at a work do three months ago), I poured a glass of champagne over his head. I still crave what I thought I had with him, but it *is* getting better. The last thing I want is to go through this again (or make someone else go through it), hence no promises of fidelity and no nosy questions if I can remember to avoid asking them. I just want to concentrate on what's fun in each relationship.

As for licking my wounds, I'm already covered in a fine film of saliva and my tongue's lost all sensation . . .

Friday 26th August

The Sailor emailed to confirm that he's coming to London, asking if I had a sofa he could crash on, or if he should make alternative arrangements. Very chivalrous, I must say, but I'd rather hoped he'd stay with a friend. I don't have a sofa, or a living room. He signed off 'Gentleman of the Realm', which made me laugh.

I should probably explain that I met him on a dating site for people with STDs. Yes, really. I read a *Cosmo* article about how these sites were safe communities for people with skin complaints down below to find love because there was no awkwardness – you both knew what each other had, straight up. No agonising about when to break the news.

I got diagnosed with HPV (human papilloma virus, which can cause warts and cervical cancer) last year and although it is very common it got me really down at the time so I thought I'd join the site and see what the fuss was about. And that's where I got chatting with the Sailor. The only downside I can see is that he has a different STD to me, which means that he has certain times when he can't have sex because it's a chronic condition that flares up occasionally.

He is a handsome, well-travelled guy in his thirties who loves sailing – hence the nickname. When I stayed with my friend up in Edinburgh we arranged to meet up and there was definite chemistry, so now I'm looking forward to spending more time with him – whatever that might involve. He's meant to be moving down south to start a master's degree and might end up in London. I suppose it's an unorthodox way to meet, but does that matter when things work out?

Porsche Boy is on a business trip to Asia but hasn't bothered to keep in touch. I haven't heard from him in a week or more. I'm wondering if I should end things with him. I'm not sure what he's after – I've met all his friends, he gets so turned on by my 'fine booty' that he comes in one minute flat, and yet I have no idea when his birthday is or anything like that and we're running out of conversation.

I miss the 'click' I thought was there when I first met him.

The other morning when I'd stayed over at his and he was frying me eggs and bacon for breakfast, I couldn't think of a single thing to say after I'd exhausted small talk about his flat and his job. So what does that leave me with, apart from some very frustrating sex?

I'm not seeing any of the boys this weekend because my friend Jess is over from the States and we're going to Notting Hill to dance our asses off at the carnival.

Tuesday August 30th

Had a great day at Notting Hill carnival yesterday with Jess. We got drunk on margaritas, danced on a little fake beach under palm trees outside the Westbourne and ate greasy, spicy chicken. A total stranger danced salsa with me in the middle of the road, and I got blisters despite my Dr Scholl's – so much for 'healthy' shoes. It took three hours to get home through the crowds, but it was definitely worth it.

When Jess and I finally got on a bus I checked my phone and lo and behold there were some nice, sexy texts from Porsche Boy. Hello stranger. He wanted to know what perfume I like, so he can get me some in duty free (woo hoo! All I asked for was a chocolate bar with weird writing on it) and then he told me to keep my legs closed till he gets back. Poor sod!

I texted back to say I was too tired right now to share my bed with any of my current lovers but he'd inspired me to have a lil' wank. He wrote back instantly saying I should think of his cock sliding deep inside me. I gave him something to think about then chucked my phone in my bag because I could tell Jess was getting bored watching me chuckling to myself.

'Are you still doing that internet dating?' she asked me, casually.

'Yes. That was one of the guys just texting.'

'*How* many men are you seeing?' she raised her eyebrows.

'Not that many, Jess, don't panic. I'm just not being serious about any of them.'

'Don't you think you're just on the rebound?'

'I don't think so . . . Anyway, even if I were, what else am I supposed to do? Sit at home looking at a photo of Pinocchio?' My phone beeped deep in my bag.

I didn't need this from Jess, especially after Samantha told me yesterday that Pinocchio thinks I'm 'unstable'.

Well, I thought, I suppose he would if what I did to his flat was anything to go by – I wasn't quite myself when collecting my things – but that was nearly six months ago, and anyway, how did my best mate Sam know about that? I suppose he must have told her, plus a few embellishments, to make himself look like the innocent victim.

'I'm having fun,' I said firmly. 'As long as I'm single, I'm free to do as I please. It's a real ego boost to have all these guys after me, they're all really sexy.' She didn't look jealous; she looked like she didn't quite believe me. Shit, is she trying to make me feel guilty? What does she know about being the centre of attention for a multitude of cute guys? She has a fantastic banker boyfriend and I can't remember her having her heart broken before. Maybe she worries that I'll never be back to my 'old self'. Maybe that's not such a bad thing. I think the things you go through just become part of your emotional make up – everyone comes with baggage, it's how you deal with it that counts. And I don't see what business it is of hers, or Pinocchio's.

I got home late and soaked my poor feet in the bath. Chubby Boy called from Edinburgh, we chatted for a bit and I told him about my day at the carnival. Then he said he was getting into bed and I should too, and I thought, 'I know where this is going, and I'm not sure I'm looking forward to it . . .' – isn't phone sex just totally naff? How are you supposed to get off with just a handset for company? He still has that killer accent though, so I let him win me over.

Man, was I surprised – what a conversation.

We started out very subtly. He even asked, 'What are you wearing?' which cracked me up. Baggy old pyjamas! He told me to take them off. Hello? I told him I don't like sleeping in the nude, and anyway he was in Scotland, so he wouldn't know if they were on or off. He said he could tell by my voice if I was lying to him. The cheeky sod, but I tell you, on the phone he's got a real authority, in a sexy, sensitive way, I mean.

He explained how he would slip my pyjamas off and stroke me slowly, then kiss my thighs and lick me . . . I just lay there holding the phone to my ear with one hand and letting the other one follow his voice down between my legs as he told me how good I tasted and how hard he was getting. I touched myself where he told me he was running his tongue, his voice in my ear, feeling myself getting turned on despite myself, giggling less. I started to get really into it. I described how I was going to lick his cock, take it into my mouth, play with his balls. I broke off to kiss him and told him to turn me over, grab me by the hips and try and push himself into me, then I sat up over him and teased him, lowering myself onto him just a little so the head of his cock just slipped into my pussy, feeling the rim of it right on the edge of me, thinking about letting him fuck me hard. I ran my finger round the lips of my cunt and told him to push me away and bend me over in front of him, then plunged two fingers in. All the time he kept talking, keeping up this mono-logue in my ear about the way we'd fucked in Edinburgh, and what I felt like inside, and I was twisting on my fingers, until I came – a really intense orgasm. His breathing got harder and faster as he heard me, and held the phone down to my pussy and mashed it with my hand so he could hear the noise it made, and the slap of my hand on my bum. I told him when he came that morning in Edinburgh he showered me with warm spunk from my neck to my thighs, and then I heard him come, too: with a loud 'Fuuuuuuck!'

So, I lost my phone sex cherry – I admit it, I get what the fuss is now. We talked for a while and he tried to get me to promise him I'd come up to Scotland to see him or go to some party in Birmingham, and I'm tempted, damn! I was meant to be keeping him at arm's length. If this is rebounding, I think I like it.

2

Horizontal Communication

AUTUMN 2005

Saturday 3rd September

I will *not* phone the Pilot. Maybe I scared him off by asking why he doesn't want a girlfriend. This constant 'out of contact' behaviour seems so odd from a guy who asked me to travel to Australia with him on our first date . . .

I know he has irregular working hours and doesn't always switch his mobile on, and he told me he's bad at communication, but I think he knows he's being rude. And here's another thing: I checked out pilot training schemes online, and yes, if you finance it yourself it takes over £50,000! No wonder he won't want to get distracted by relationships if this much moolah is at stake. And I'm not sure I could spend another three years dating someone who is basically a student – a very skint, very busy student. Besides, I fancy him enough in his work uniform now, so if he were a commercial pilot I wouldn't be able to let him out of the house without making him give me a quick seeing to in the hall. Except that it's never quick with him . . .

Hmmm, yeah, where was I? That's what I'm afraid of, my mind and my heart running away with me and making me vulnerable again. I'm still looking for the right one; that's why I'm dating all these men simultaneously and getting to know them, but when you have all these expectations of a person, you want them perfect, you want yourself perfect ... Maybe I should give up on the Pilot if he's essentially disqualified himself. After all, the higher you climb the further you fall.

Tuesday 13th September

I saw him for the first time yesterday in my evening class (I'm working on my career, as well as my love life) and he was half an hour late. He looks like a black Brad Pitt, only with bigger, nicer and more sensitive lips. He's tall with incredible soft green eyes, a little beard, multicoloured dreadlocks and caramel skin. I took in every inch of him: I was even lusting after the flash of hairless skin at the top of his ankles, just above his socks. I wanted to run my tongue between his combats and those socks and taste his skin ...

I can imagine his beautiful face on top of mine, waking up next to it ... I want his lips on the lips between my legs, his tongue darting out to touch my clit. I can picture his cock straining against the material of those Calvins, and maybe the head of it peeking out, aching to be inside me. I'm getting wet and want to rub myself against him, find his fingers.

I imagine his dick pushing the material of his pants aside and sliding up my thigh towards my pussy. I feel the urge to just keep pushing against him, to push him inside me, open up and just suck him in. My thighs are slick with my own wetness, the soft head of his penis follows the trail and I open my legs just a bit more.

Our mouths are sucking, licking, stuck together. I throw my head back and he grazes my neck with his teeth and licks and sucks my chin, my ear lobes, my neck until I squirm and laugh and pull his head away from me by his dreads. He drops his head, licking the tops of my breasts, teasing my nipples, forcing his knee between my thighs. I can feel his soft, scratchy shin and his heavy, muscular thigh on top of me, his chest so close to my mouth, huge and hard with erect, small dark nipples.

He grabs my wrists, spreads me out on the bed and slowly inches upwards, and I want him and I don't stop him and lift my pelvis up towards his cock. He looks me in the eye and kisses me, then slides slowly into me, right up to the hilt. Then he pulls out again, almost all the way. He thrusts again and I don't want him to stop . . .

Well, it gives me something to think about in class.

Wednesday 14th September

The Pilot pissed me off today. I finally got through to him and invited him to a work party but he said he didn't want to come because it was in a 'dodgy' part of London and it would be late, oh and 'it's not his scene'. Hello?

So, he has no interest in my work or life. Can't you hear the alarm bells starting to ring? He went to Soho Pride with me and that's not exactly his scene either, *and* I almost got beaten up by a nasty French lesbian who I caught jumping the loo queue. Isn't that 'dodgy' enough for him?

I told him that he didn't get raped by rampant gay boys in Soho and he won't get mugged by stoned black men at this party. What a wimp. Porsche Boy's no better. He can 'squeeze me in' just once a week, and tells me to keep my legs together the rest of the time. He seems to have misunderstood the situation.

Friday 23rd September

I'm finally meeting the Sailor again this weekend. He's in London to look at universities for his master's degree, and I'm flat-sitting for Samantha while she's away on holiday with her bloke, which means I will have a sofa to offer him. He doesn't want us to plan too much of the weekend, just let it unfold and see what we fancy doing. Be nice to get to know him better, and maybe fuck his highly intelligent brains out if the chemistry I felt when I met him in Edinburgh is anything to go by!

Sunday 25th September

After spending twenty-three hours in the Sailor's company, I'm hooked. Yesterday I made him lunch at Samantha's and we went for a long walk in the park and then along by the canal, talking and laughing. Later we met up with Canada Boy and his mate from Brazil at the pub for a drink (did I mention that the Sailor speaks fluent Portuguese?) Canada Boy recommended a restaurant and we said goodbye to them and had a lovely dinner with more wine and more talk, covering everything from religion to our parents and grandparents' relationships, to our experiences of travelling in Thailand. We hadn't even kissed.

Then we went on to a club. I wanted to get him on the dance floor and check his moves and his confidence, but it was fairly quiet when we got there. So after a glass of bubbly for me, some beer and a couple of smokes for him, we began dancing as the floor finally started filling up. He's a great mover, although it's a pity about the cigarettes. He says he's trying to give up, but that's what they all say. Reminds me a bit of Pinocchio, although I put up with his habit.

Things got more touchy-feely with the Sailor and eventually he kissed me. Finally feeling his lips on mine was fantastic. He moved behind me and held my wrists, and I tipped my head back against him, super-aware of his lips by my ear, and his broad chest. We went back to Samantha's flat.

He went outside for a last smoke and in a mad desire for adventure I climbed up one floor on the scaffolding outside. He followed me and we stood there looking out and kissing. It'd been raining and I was barefoot, loving the cool damp on my sore dancing feet.

We ended up in the bedroom, and he kept up the stroking and kissing and gently pulled my top off. I was still thinking we might just end up falling asleep and I didn't want to look like I desperately didn't want that to happen, so I wouldn't take my bra off (I think I thought that was reverse psychology or something). He let his hands wander up under my skirt and I gasped and realised just how turned on I was.

I was very, very wet. He teased my clit and entered me with his fingers and then I wanted his cock inside me badly, even though I knew we couldn't because it was the wrong 'time of the month' for him and his STD. It's bizarre that whole advertising campaigns are dedicated towards treating cold sores as long as they're on someone's face, yet when the offending herpes virus takes up residence below one's belly button, it's a whole different ball game shrouded in shame and taboos. I could see the frustration in his face, but he went on rubbing and probing me with his fingers and eventually went down on me, his fingers still deep in my pussy.

He went on licking me relentlessly, moving his fingers in me, until it got too much and I squirmed and stroked his face so he'd stop. I lay there in his arms with this weird sense of having come, but still needing more: I just wanted to touch him and feel him inside me, but he kept his boxers on and insisted he was fine. 'I'm not eighteen any more,' he said, and I could feel the heat and hardness of him through the material.

The Sailor dozed off, eventually, and in the morning he made me French toast and did all the washing up. It all just felt really relaxed and I don't think I would have said no to him and his soft skin, toned body, blue eyes. He even thanked me for trusting him. I thanked him for his generosity, his warmth and of course, that orgasm . . .

Of course, now I want him so much I can barely see straight. Since then he's been texting me, telling me he loves the taste of me and how much he wants to make love to me. Chubby just texted to ask if I'd been up to anything exciting this weekend. Do you think he *really* wants to know?

Monday 10th October

I sat next to black Brad Pitt (BBP) in class today. He smells of shower gel and deodorant. It's like you can feel every muscle without even touching him. I wanted to reach out and touch those broad shoulders, unveil that muscly back and scrape his dreadlocks to one side to kiss his silky, brown neck.

He came for a drink with a gang of us afterwards, and kept buying me rounds. Unfortunately BBP isn't a great conversationalist. If he were a bit more confident (or possibly older – he's only twenty-four) or cocky then, my God, I couldn't hold off. But maybe it's a good thing he's a bit shy, because then he'd be more faithful. On the *other* hand, I don't care about that, do I? I just want his body, not his eternal troth.

I gave him a little shoulder massage when he said he felt a bit stiff, and his body felt as good as it looked. I think he enjoyed it. It turns out he used to run a lot, and his legs were certainly a testament to that when I *accidentally* brushed them under the table with my own. I guess there's no way anything could really happen with us. He is far too beautiful to fancy me, and comes across a bit too stupid for me to really fancy him . . . I mean, give me David Beckham any day, but make sure he keeps his mouth shut! I'm a bad girl – I wouldn't respect him enough. Definitely not fair to try and pull him, unless of course he made all the moves and I was unable to resist . . .

Bad Sienna.

Monday 17th October

I was just having a quiet little wank, thinking about the Sailor. It's mind-blowing and such a turn on to really want someone having been so close . . . but no cigar. I can't wait till we really have sex. He's been texting up a storm, telling me he's found a place in the West Country (he won't be in London for his masters after all), saying he would come to see me if he could get a flight, but . . . Nothing was promised, and he wasn't in touch again so I assume he couldn't find one. What's wrong with using a train if he really wanted to see me? So I'm a bit sad, thinking of sleeping next to him and waking up to see his smile, those incredible eyes. Even though he's a smoker he didn't snore, and his skin was soooo soft.

I can't believe I didn't even get to see his dick.

He says he's going to top his last performance next time though. No shit!

Saturday 22nd October

OK, now that's asking for it. BBP got my phone number from one of the other girls on my evening course and phoned me on Friday night when I was minding my own business and trying to sort something out with the computer. He said he was 'sort of in the area' and wondered what I was doing. Then he asked me out for a drink. I couldn't say no.

He picked me up and we went to a venue with a salsa night.

At first I hardly recognised him when I walked up to his car – he's not much of gentleman so he didn't get out – with a red bandana obscuring his dreads he looked like a very tanned Captain Jack Sparrow. I was overexcited, but the conversation didn't exactly flow until we started playing a drinking game called 'I have never'.

You say something you've never done and if the other person *has*, they have to drink. You start out slowly, with things like 'I've never been to Uruguay' then move on to 'I've never had a period' (him – so I had to drink) and 'I've never slept with a girl' (me – so he had to drink). Aaaand you get quite drunk, quite quickly, depending on how adventurous you've been.

Halfway through I got a text message from Porsche Boy, dumping me:

'Hey you.'
Told you he never uses my name.
'I feel like we've lost touch recently. Blame it on work etc . . .'
His, I guess?
'But I think we're heading in different directions.'
Yup, and we're both heading away from your bed.
'Anyway, I'm confused.'
Doesn't sound like it.
'Guess we say gbye?'

And I just about managed to message back, 'So I'm dumped by text? Boo hoo ;) I'm out dancing!' because what else can you say, really? Plus I couldn't say I cared, not when I had BBP smiling at me, maybe looking a bit worried about me getting texts at one a. m.

I finally managed to pull BBP up to dance with me; he was a

bit embarrassed because he doesn't have a clue how to salsa, but I got him to improvise and then snuggled myself against his chest and hips. Our faces were about an inch away from each other. I felt his breath on my cheek and his strong leg between my thighs and suddenly we were kissing. I wish I hadn't been so drunk, but it was really overdue. The conversation had been a little bit one-sided and all I wanted was to rip his clothes off, so kissing came as a lovely relief. His lips were so soft and he was such a great kisser.

We ended up leaving half the wine abandoned on the table because it was so sickly sweet, and then he drove me home. More kissing. I jumped out of the car, waved and went straight in. I was half expecting him to ask if he could come up, but I'm glad he didn't. I was far too drunk.

I forgot all about Porsche Boy till I was checking my phone this morning. That's the way to break up! I suppose my plan worked like it's supposed to: we both got something without losing anything. Sorted.

Monday 24th October

No word from the Pilot. Did he crash? I mean, I didn't contact him because I was so annoyed about the party but then I read something in the paper about a flying instructor and another pilot crashing near an airfield, and I know it's not his airfield, but it still made me uneasy. I resisted texting him because I was sure I was setting myself up for another heartache, like we were overdue for an 'I like you, but . . . ' conversation.

I'm sure he's fine. It's just that loads of little things are making me think of him. I need to stop feeling responsible for other people all the time. I mean, he can call me, right? But he obviously doesn't want to.

BBP was up till two a. m. texting me, wanting to feel my lips again. The feeling is mutual.

Wednesday 26th October

I miss the Sailor and the Pilot. Maybe I'll just tell them about each other, so they don't feel like they're under pressure and then I can restrict myself to just two men for the rest of my life, and make both those relationships emotionally meaningful and sexually fulfilling and they can have all the time they need to get on with their studies while I'm busy with the other guy. And if I'm bored I can go flying with one and sailing with the other. And if I want to go off on my own they can both look after the kids.

Think that would work?

Monday 7th November

I did it. Twice. I did the deed with BBP! I'd cooked for him and he was late – at first I almost felt like some sad little housewife, preparing food for an ungrateful husband – it all seemed a bit domestic – but my heart melted when he insisted on saying grace and we had a lovely time eating the meal. We went into my bedroom to chill out for a bit with some music and TV. He still wasn't saying much, but I tried not to let that bother me.

I offered him a massage, first his back, and then the demanding little so-and-so insisted I do his legs as well, but I told him that'd only happen if he reciprocated. I made him take his shirt off and got my massage oil. His body was everything I'd imagined, and the colour of chocolate milkshake. No spots, only a small scar near his nipple, above his heart, where he told me he'd been stabbed. Yes, really. He was trying to defend a mate who was being attacked and three guys jumped on him, one with a knife.

So I'm moving along his legs, his trousers still on, just pushing them up as I go, but um, how do you massage someone's thighs? I did my best. Then he rolled over onto his back. I was trying not to feel a little bit used. Where was *my* massage? He might have fallen asleep or left before it was my turn (it's happened before, don't ask). I mean, we hadn't kissed since our date in the salsa club.

This time we weren't drunk. When he started to touch my back I felt the wetness start to flood. I pulled off my top and unhooked my bra so he could smooth the oil right up to my neck. His hands were amazing – big and a bit rough, but well shaped and cared for. He has small calluses from weightlifting, but his fingernails are immaculate. Lying there, the thought that he might have manicures flickered through my head and made me smile. Nah, I think he must just be naturally perfect.

When he put his hands side by side on my spine they covered my waist, warmed every fibre in my muscles. He was so thorough that I was beginning to wonder if he really *did* see this as just a massage, but when he started on my calves I think my giggling and gasping gave me away. I never knew an oily thumb in the back of my knee could be so erotic.

A part of me could still barely believe it was happening. Usually when I fancy someone this much they just don't want to know. He took my breath away just walking into the classroom, and now he was in my bedroom, wanting me.

He rolled me onto my back again and came closer. I could feel his dreads against my skin. Then he lay next to me with his arm around me and looked into my eyes. He's so beautiful. He pushed my hair out of my face and kissed me tenderly on the lips.

We started to kiss and roll together, fingernails trailing over skin. He kissed and sucked my neck, then pushed his hand gently into my bra and caressed my nipple. More teasing, kissing and rolling and we had our hands in each other's pants, then I was on top of him and tugging his trousers off. The tip of his penis was peeking out of the top of his Calvins, just like in my fantasy.

I inched my way down his stomach, pressing my lips on his belly and took him in my mouth. I was pleased with his taste. His girth was quite generous but thankfully it wasn't the monster I'd feared. A little salty, like pre-cum, but not unpleasant. I tried not to let him come, kept it brief and then moved up next to him again. He was tickling my clit with one finger, and asked me what I wanted him to do.

I asked him to lick me, and he gave me this most gorgeous expression, then slowly, slowly went down on me. He knelt on the floor and buried his face between my thighs, sucked my clitoris till I came, his lips enveloping it.

I hugged and kissed him then pulled him up on top of me. I pulled his boxer shorts off, grabbed a condom and peeled it on him, then rolled him on his back and straddled him. He looked like an angel with his dreadlocks spread out on my pillow, and his green eyes looking up at me.

His cock felt great inside me . . . Everything was mad and amazing after that, like we were trying every possible position. It was all totally natural, even though there is no page in the *Kama Sutra* where the man is sitting on the edge of the bed and penetrating the woman as she hangs away backwards, balancing herself with one hand on the floor and one on his foot. We were both dripping with sweat by the time he came, and I had to give him a towel to dry himself off.

I lay on his chest and he wrapped his arm round me, stroking my back as he drifted off, then waking up and peering at me from under those long curly lashes, then drifting off again. After a few hours we were both awake; it was dark, and we fucked again, finishing with him behind me, grasping my hair.

I wasn't sure if he would want to stay the whole night. It was still pretty early, and he seemed tired while I had things to potter round and do before I went to sleep. Some girl rang him, and he ignored his phone. I asked if it was his girlfriend, and he looked shocked: 'Why would I have sex with you if I had a girlfriend?' I just thought it best to ask – why *would* he tell me if he had one? After all he knows nothing about my love life. I just don't want to be the reason for someone else getting hurt.

He had a quick shower and then I went to close the door downstairs behind him. 'I'll have such a stupid grin on my face in class tomorrow,' I told him as he kissed me goodbye. Afterwards I wondered where this is going. As I expected, he's phenomenal in bed, but a bit quiet and either moody or shy out of it. Wonder what he'll be like in our class tonight.

Tuesday 8th November

This morning I had a text from Pinocchio.

'How are you?'

I hate it when he pretends everything is nice and normal. We both know how it ended, and there he is, telling Samantha I'm unstable.

Now I'm wondering if I should call his mum again, because I miss her – we really hit it off. Normally she hates his girlfriends. You don't just lose one person when you break up. My violent first boyfriend had ten younger brothers and sisters who treated me like Madonna every time I walked in the door, which is more than could be said for him. Losing them hurt, but so did my bruises. I might write about that one day, but not on a day when Pinocchio's disconcerted me.

I realised the other day that a lot of the reason I get so low is that I find things from my past and project them onto new situations. So if the Pilot doesn't call it reminds me of Pinocchio not calling when I so desperately needed his reassurance after our break-up. I suppose it's just a bad habit. Be nice to talk to one of my lovers about it, but that'd be baggage. And I don't do baggage, do I?

I did see BBP in my evening class yesterday too, but it was a bit awkward. I'd just had a bad phone call with my landlord – my flatmate wants to move out and I haven't found a replacement yet – and was trying to concentrate on what the teacher was saying, while being aware of the fact that I was wearing the same t-shirt BBP had peeled off me, and he was wearing the same pair of trousers that I'd been impatiently tugging off less than twenty-four hours ago. I looked at that sliver of exposed skin on his ankle again, and remembered wanting to lick it, and getting my chance the night before, and remembered what his face looked like in the semi darkness of my room, just as he was about to sink his lips onto my clit.

I had to leave as soon as the class was over to get home and audition a potential new flatmate, but BBP beat me out of the door and I caught up with him at the bottom of the stairs. Paranoid Sienna suddenly thought he was trying to avoid me – did he think I'd kicked him out last night, or was he just trying to stop me getting the wrong idea about him, in case I thought he cared? Paranoid Sienna was way off the mark – turns out he was just worried about the place where he'd parked in case he got clamped, although of course I'd blathered out an explanation about the new flatmate before he could tell me that. He offered me a lift.

In his car we listened to 50 Cent. He knows all the words. He's a rapper himself, on the quiet, and I listened to some of his stuff last night – it was pretty good, although I don't know the first thing about rap.

He is, in a way, so foreign, so male, and so full of hidden tension and attitude. A bit of an enigma. There's so much going on in his eyes – a quick spark of passion, a lot of thoughts that never get spoken. Yesterday in my bed he looked like a huge lion, stretching and relaxing, then he was so tender too. I find it hard to follow his accent sometimes because it's such a mixture of Northern and pretend Cockney, and he has this low voice with cool, lazy diction which intrigues me even when the meaning of his words doesn't always get from my ear to my brain. That might go both ways. He is eager to brush up on his language skills, but when he asked for a translation and I told him the German word for traffic, *Verkehr*, he thought I'd said, 'Fuck here.' He seemed shocked at my outrageous 'suggestion' and it took a while to convince him that I didn't want us to do it in the car while we were stuck in slow-moving traffic – or was he just winding me up? I think we're losing a few jokes somewhere. I also think he covers up his intelligence too well, although I don't know why he bothers. I hardly know a thing about him but he acts like he's from the 'hood although his adoptive parents are well-off and he is good at languages and quite arty.

I opened up a little, even though I was trying not to get too 'heavy' and push him away. I hinted at what had happened with Pinocchio and confessed how vulnerable that had left me. He listened and seemed to care, but stayed silent, so I went on and told him I don't always like to be teased, especially when I am feeling fragile, and then I worried that he thought I was criticising his sense of humour. It seems like the less you say, the more you find out about people. Maybe that's a lesson I should take to heart.

I touched his neck and back and he asked me if he felt stiff, and I had to fight off the urge to give him a pat on the crotch and quote Julia Roberts in *Pretty Woman*, 'Not yet, but it's got potential,' but the atmosphere in the car was all wrong for that kind of quip. There's something a little awkward about being with him, mixed with a really quiet intimacy. I know it's all going *in*, but I don't know what he thinks because there's no feedback from him, so I rattle on.

As he pulled up outside my house I kissed him on the side of the mouth, but he didn't pull me in for a snog. Why is he playing it so cool? I opened the door and turned back and kissed him more firmly. He could have held on to me but he didn't.

The potential flatmate was waiting for me. We got on really well, so fingers crossed she can move in as soon as old flatmate moves out.

Friday 18th November

I cancelled an interview for a job today. I know I don't like the place where I am now, but this would just have been a stopgap to get me out of there – better if I put up with my boss for a few more months and wait for the right job to come along, where I have a chance to really shine instead of using up my creativity fabricating excuses for my boss.

It might be a strength or a weakness, but I never expect people to change or stop making the same mistakes. My boss called me into his office the other day to talk about my 'job satisfaction' and I mentioned his last-minute, 'Oh, Sienna? Could you just photocopy this 400-page file and pop it on my desk? And add an index while you're at it?' trick and of course he promised to 'be more thoughtful in the future' but I doubt it.

It's just the same with the Pilot. He won't contact me for weeks on end; he told me he wasn't good at 'keeping in touch' with his ex-girlfriend. I'd rather walk away. When I was little I wasted a lot of time forgiving my dad for things he did, instead of seeing him for the person he really is. It took a long time, but I got less tolerant, and maybe that makes me unpleasant to deal with sometimes. And maybe that intolerance and unforgiving attitude means that sometimes, when I'm walking away, my heart is heavy with regret.

People are attracted by my light, sparkly side, the side that wants everyone to come to the party and be looked after, but I'm scared that they'll be horrified when they see the discoloured and rusty flipside of the coin. The side that makes me paranoid about BBP and the Pilot. Sometimes I need to rein my thoughts and feelings back in and look at them in a different light: if a girlfriend doesn't phone, how do I know that it's because 'she hates me'? Why should BBP's reserve mean that he doesn't understand? He might get it after all.

Then again, sometimes you just know. People go off you; they don't feel the same way; they don't want to be the thing you want them to be.

Saturday 26th November

Lonesome. I went out with some girlfriends last night, had one cocktail and started crying about Pinocchio. Way to go, Sienna.

I got a text from the Sailor saying he can't come down for the weekend after all because he has to study. I was quite upbeat about it – hey, I'm not his girlfriend, and I'll just see him when-ever. That's how this thing works.

Less good was the parcel from the Pilot containing a DVD I'd lent him and no note. I'd asked for it back, and I was quite brief with him on the phone because I was so fed up with him being distant, but it's not what I'd call closure. I'm not going to let it get to me. At least he's not lying, although even Porsche Boy managed to be more direct with a drunken text at one a. m. ('we're headed in different directions' – yes, you to Boringland in a Porsche, me in search of fresh adventures on my skateboard).

No answer to the big 'WHY?' though. I knew deep down we weren't suited and that the timing was off, and I bet he did too, but nothing's going to weasel that out of him. If only he weren't so cute and such a good lover, I might not care so much . . .

Canada Boy's been quiet too.

Monday 28th November

Tonight was just odd. Wild and horny and a bit confusing.

I caught up with BBP after class when he was ambling down the street chatting on his mobile, and pulled his hood up over his head from behind. He smiled and after some chit-chat we ended up in a restaurant nearby. He said he was tired and we didn't talk much, but we shared each other's food a little, and he said he'd like to come back to mine.

I put an arm round him on the bus and he stroked my hand, and we just sat there chewing our gum in silence, him with his headphones on – a bit weird given that his iPod was dead. I asked him why and he said he didn't know where else to put them, which made me laugh, although I wasn't sure if he meant it to be funny.

When we got to mine he refused a drink and followed me up to my room, saying, 'You could have tidied up,' when my room was immaculate, or at least, not bad for me, but I didn't know if it was a joke or not. Then he stretched out on the bed looking sleepy and I joined him, trying to make a little flirty conversation to provoke him out of his lethargy. I tried to tell him about the film I'd seen the night before but somehow he interpreted that as me having just come back from the country where it was set. The conversation just kept getting weirder.

The chat meandered a little and he told me, 'I don't like girls.' What? OK, this I had to know. 'Why not? What do you mean?' 'Cos most of them are sluts.' I was shocked – what would he think if he knew? How the fuck does he define what a 'slut' is? But I decided to keep the tone light and asked him why he liked me, given that I was a girl. 'But you're Sienna!' he grinned, cutely.

We started kissing and stroking. I don't 'get' him, but he's so beautiful to look at that it makes me happy just to be around him. Communication is better when we stop talking. We lay face to face, him stroking and lightly scratching my back the way I like it, me trailing my fingers across his neck, over his biceps and down his back.

Things got more heated and my clothes started coming off till I was lying naked on him and he was still in his boxers and shirt. I get so turned on just seeing him touch me, and the contrast between our skin and hair, and seeing my fingers on his pecs. His body is the sweetest surprise. Clothed, he looks almost skinny, even if you can make out his pecs through his shirt, but naked he's powerfully built, even with a tiny belly and an adorable butt that makes me think his trousers would probably fit me too.

After a while, we don't seem to have any difficulty understanding each other. In bed he's vocal, lets me know what he wants ('Sit on my face and let me lick you') and understands what I'm asking for intuitively. When we lose our clothes we lose all that awkwardness and misunderstanding, and we meet on the same level of pure lust, revelling in each other's bodies.

When he reaches into my knickers he doesn't fumble around, but goes straight to the sweet spot and touches me exactly right. I nearly came but held back and told him I wanted him to lick my clit, knowing he would anyway, but also knowing that it turns him on to hear me ask for it. He moved down my body, looking up at me with his big, beautiful eyes then slowly slipping a finger in and out of me as he sucked and kissed me till I came.

I pulled him up to my face again so our bodies were pressed together, and kissed him, letting him feel the little post-orgasmic shivers that were running through me and letting him know how good he was. I reached down to his shorts which were damp from my wetness, and pulled his cock out. He watched me as I blew him until I got impatient and reached for a condom because I had to have him inside me.

When we fuck he has a way of combining roughness with courtesy, so he'll crush me in his arms and pull my hair to hold me still, but never ram into me with his dick – which has considerable girth – careful not to hurt me. When he starts to move I get greedy and want him to roger me senseless, and he teases me by slowing, saying he has to stop himself coming too soon, telling me I'm too tight. It sounds so corny and dirty typing it up now, but in the moment it sounds like he means it, and he kept going till I finally came and so did he.

He pulled the duvet over us, hugging me and stroking my arm lazily, then fell asleep on my breast, snoring. I got up carefully and went to the bathroom, hoping my new flatmate wouldn't catch me walking naked across the landing, then returned to find BBP still sleeping, looking so fucking adorable that I wanted to take a flying leap from the door and cuddle him. 'You're just like a baby, all you want to do is sleep, eat and suck my tits.' He laughed, eyes opening a crack: 'What's wrong with that?' I slipped under the duvet next to him and he pushed a hand into my pubes, finding my clit and rubbing it in slow, firm circles. I felt him hardening against my thigh and pushed my pelvis up against his hand, wanting more.

This time I crouched on all fours with him behind me, rocking and slapping himself against my behind, one hand teasing my clit until I came, then turned, stripped the condom off him and took him into my mouth again. Just before he came I pulled back so he spurted all over my breasts and belly.

A minute or two later he was asleep, his perfect, edible bum sticking out of the duvet. I curled up in the crook of his body and felt very fulfilled and happy.

Monday 5th December

BBP stayed away from our evening class today. I have no idea if he was avoiding me (probably not) or just busy or tired, as always. I texted him to ask if he wanted to work on our presentations together, and he replied, dumbly, 'What presentations?'

Tuesday 13th December

I caved in and texted the Pilot. No reply.

BBP phoned at tea time to tell me he was tired and going to sleep. OK, whatever. I suggested he rang on Sunday if he wanted to go swimming or something, but he never did. Christ knows what's going on in his head, all I know is he won't share it with me. Why call when you have nothing to say and no desire to arrange a date? I am confused.

I know I'm supposed to be Sienna the libertine with no strings attached, but there's some chemical that makes people fall 'in love' once they've exchanged sweat and saliva. I'm confusing myself most of all. Why isn't hot sex and a hot body rolling around on top of you enough?

I'm starting to really care for BBP and I know we wouldn't work as a couple, I just know that. We haven't talked about 'us' and I know it's one of those conversations boys don't start, but I'm afraid.

I'm afraid he will fall in love with me and catch me out, realising it's just sex for me.

I'm afraid he sees it as just sex and he's seeing other girls, and then I'll feel rejected and hurt.

I'm afraid he'll be angry about me seeing other guys and he'll hit me, but I don't know why – that fear is nothing to do with him or the way he acts to me. Where did I get this fear? Bastard first boyfriend? Why am I projecting it onto BBP?

None of these fears add up. It doesn't make any sense.

Thursday 15th December

Forgive me, boss, for I have sinned:

- I have been writing my blog during hours when I should have been at your disposal.
- I have bought chocolate bars with the petty cash.
- I have used your stamps to send a few letters and nicked blank CDs and stationery.
- I have used expensive printer cartridges to print pictures of me and my lover.
- I have snuck off on interviews for other jobs, having told you I went to view a flat/feed my friend's cat/see the doctor.
- I have been watching telly and being lazy while you're out of the office.

- I hid your biscuits when you told me I'd bought unhealthy food for the office. And then I ate them myself.
- I have used the company phone for private calls.
- I have used the fax machine to apply for other jobs.
- I would have no qualms about having a lover round for an afternoon fuck if no one were here.
- I have had a wank on the office sofa, and then answered the phone without washing my hands.
- I've eaten stuff from the fridge that wasn't mine.
- I have flirted with your accountant.

However, I am prepared to stop sinning if:

- You stop booking cabs for family members on the office account.
- You stop asking me for petty cash you don't return or provide receipts for.
- You stop 'running errands' on office time.
- You give me proper excuses to use when your wife calls.
- You manage to go to the loo for less than fifteen minutes at a time when you get an important phone call, and don't pop out for 'quick breaks' which take a minimum of two hours and involve switching your mobile off.
- You stop blaming me for your own mistakes.
- You stop stealing stamps for your private letters.
- You stop eating my fruit.
- You stop giving me confusing instructions and agree not to save the things you want me to do till the last minute when I want to go home.
- You stop expecting me to read your mind.

Friday 16th December

I think my tryst with BBP has reached the stage where 'just sex' doesn't cut it any more. I think I won't call him again. I know it's not 'going anywhere' and there's a tension that stops it being just a carefree sexual affair. I worry about my sanity.

While I was at my friend Nicola's flat for her Christmas party last night he phoned me four times and hardly said anything. Each time I had to run out into the freezing garden to take his call because of bad mobile reception inside, and the others wondered why he didn't just come to the party. He didn't want to. Instead I decided to go home early and he came round at midnight when I was wrapped up in my silky nightgown, and we fell into bed.

Since none of the guys I've been seeing since Pinocchio have been my boyfriend, I've not introduced many of them to friends – not that I don't want to, but often I just don't see them enough myself or it could be awkward.

Samantha met the Pilot at Gay Pride in the summer, Canada Boy knows a few of my friends (mostly because he's a friend, not a lover, and we are very comfortable with each other), and a couple of my girlfriends met BBP in November, when he was out with his friends and I was out with mine.

In all the time we spent together last night, BBP only said five words that weren't about my clit or my breasts or my pussy. I'd wanted him there badly, wanting to lay to rest some of the awkwardness after we last fucked, and once again the communication problems fell away and we were devouring each other in bed. Afterwards he fell asleep again, although his breathing seemed too fast and I wondered if he were just shutting me out and pretending. I couldn't relax and lay there watching him, knowing in my heart that this was going to have to be the last time, and that it would be so hard to let him go. Even though he was asleep there seemed to be something awkward in the atmosphere. I woke him up with a blow job this morning all the same.

But then he left without having breakfast, telling me he didn't want to get a parking ticket, and making me feel like a fool for bringing a tray from the kitchen. I saw him sitting in his car outside the house, unwrapping a packet of his favourite sweets that I'd given him at the door as an early Christmas present. He was still there fifteen minutes later so I rang him to ask if everything was OK and he asked me what I was going on about because he was driving to work. I checked again and his car was gone. Why didn't he just tell me what he'd been doing?

He wished me a merry Christmas when he left, with a kiss on the lips. Merry Christmas indeed. At least I got into work on time.

3

The Soulless Soulmate

WINTER 2005/2006

Saturday 17th December

I had a Christmas shopping frenzy today – trying to get everything done before I fly to my mum's – and ended up in a street
in Covent Garden that always triggers a memory that makes
me smile. I woke up in a flat there once – the morning after my
first visit to a fetish club – you could say I plunged in headfirst.

I'd gone with a group of open-minded friends who weren't
really into the scene and we were just planning to have a laugh.
I wore a PVC top and a rubber skirt – just some cheap stuff I'd
picked up in Camden Market – high boots and lots of eyeliner.
And underwear, which shows how much I know!

We got a lot more than we bargained for. I think I knew that
'fetish' can mean just about anything, but when you see 'everything' laid out in front of you, well, it's a bit overwhelming.
There was one older guy with a perm who wore nothing but a
pair of sheer women's panties and heels.

We were sticking together on the dance floor, dancing but
goggling at everything that was going on, the little sub/dom
fantasies being acted out. Someone was being flogged next door
(you could hear the slaps and howls over the music). Some of
the women had more cellulite than rubber, and some of the men

had more hair and piercings than PVC. I didn't really plan to end up being part of the floor show, but then this tall, gorgeous boy in leather trousers with a dog collar and leash round his neck came up to me.

I don't remember much small talk, only that he was happy for me to snap his lead and make him call me mistress. We danced for a while, as I held the lead, giving it the occasional jerk to keep him on his toes, then went upstairs to the play area. It was dark, it smelled sweaty, and people were horny.

My slave kissed me and pulled me towards him, his back to the wall. I felt a hand tracing up my skirt towards my bum, then two hands fiddling with my knickers and trying to stroke my crotch from behind. It was nice for a few seconds, like a sexy dream in the dark, and then I realised it was two strangers behind me as *well* as my slave and I freaked out a little and asked them to stop. They backed off and my slave and I moved on, me tugging on his lead.

We found a shower stall for some privacy, and it turned out that he was naked under those leather pants, but I was worried about the shower head turning on and us getting soaked, so we stumbled into the toilets. There was a queue: a gimp in full rubber with a tube sticking out of his mask, a few trannies, women with peek-a-boo rubber bras, suspenders and no knickers, a guy with more piercings round his anus and balls than I had in my ears . . .

Finally a stall was free. My slave pushed me up against the partition and knelt in front of me, pushed my knickers aside and my skirt up and licked me. He gazed up at me like a puppy, begging me to come in his face, but even though I was really horny I don't think I came – it was too bright and too weird. Also I was worried about the queue outside. I must have sort of faked it, but he was probably disappointed I didn't squirt him in the eye!

We went back to his flat as the sun was coming up, and, after he'd pulled out some clothes pegs and put them on his nipples, and then, almost putting me off my stroke, pulled the skin round his balls tight and clipped those too, we fucked. Unfortunately the clothes pegs weren't as great for me as they were for him – here's a tip, having wooden clothes pegs repeatedly prodded into your crotch isn't everyone's kink – but he went down on me till I was squirming, and then we fell asleep. We had breakfast in the café downstairs, and he gave me his card. He was a naked slave butler at parties. I can't remember if I called him again. I wonder if he offers a gift-wrapping service? It's the only way I'm going to get all my parcels done in time.

Sunday 18th December

Silence from BBP. I suppose I can't say this is a disaster. He doesn't seem to care that I've pulled back, which I should be happy about, but my head and my heart are a mess. My friend Lucy gave me a pep talk last night (she asked about BBP and I told her all about my recent confused feelings). She has this theory that you shouldn't go out trying to pull, but the right guy will just present himself when you *don't* need him. It's like you have to trick fate – 'Hah! Fooled you! I was lonely after all!' It's easy for her to say that as she's had a boyfriend she's been complaining about for five years, but to some extent she's got a point. Even if I'm trying not to be serious with these men, I get upset when it goes wrong and I don't need that.

A new job would be nice though. And a new boss. How does work just manage to get worse in the festive season? Why doesn't peace and good will extend to harassed office workers with idiot bosses?

Monday 19th December

How can having so much fun make you feel so bad? Yesterday Canada Boy took me to a big Christmas party at a club. The theme was Studio 54, and they had people in costume: hippies with big fake spliffs, girls in short psychedelic dresses and even some rollergirls. I should have brought my skates. There was a band and we got hammered on free drinks, and that's when we discovered the chocolate fountain. Just at the point where you're so drunk you don't care if you look like a total pig and get dripping brown sticky stuff all over your clothes. I had so much I had to run to the loo to be sick, and then Canada Boy tried to snog me when I came out, and all I wanted was something to take the taste away. I grabbed a profiterole off a passing tray instead.

Samuel L. Jackson was there so I made Canada Boy dance with me in front of him like a loon and then we disappeared behind a curtain for a bit of a snog. We went home separately and all today's been a massive comedown. Too much chocolate?

Not sure why I don't want to fuck Canada Boy – he looked great, he dances like a demon and I feel completely comfortable with him. Maybe I'm just a hypocrite because I don't want someone who thinks he'll only be happy with at least two girl-friends. I don't want to do this for ever.

Friday 23rd December

Merry Bitchmas everybody.

I went out for a drink with Samantha at one of our favourite bars last night. We haven't had much of a chance to catch up, and I was really looking forward to it, but one cocktail in we somehow touched on the subject of Pinocchio.

She decided to break some news to me. Because it was Christmas.

'Sienna, about him . . . '

She looked uncomfortable, and a little bit impatient.

'Pinocchio? You still see him? But you said you didn't talk to him any more.'

'Well Sienna, I do, I always got on really well with him and his friends.'

'You said you were more interested in being friends with me.' God, now I sound like a five year old.

'I didn't want you to get upset.'

'I'm upset now. I'm more upset because you sodding well lied to me,' my throat felt sore and scratchy and my voice was rising.

'Look, I met him at the same time you first met him – and you know we were friends too.' She sounded like she was trying to justify herself. The bastard. He pisses on my life then he moves on and takes my best friend with him. Cunt!

'Oh, don't try and pretend it's OK. I can't believe you lied to me! I asked you! And you lied!' I'd started to cry now, but tried hard to keep it in. I didn't want her to notice just how upset I was so she'd get her confirmation of how 'unstable' I still was about him. Anyway, who was I to tell Samantha whom she could be friends with?

She seemed really cold to me and eager to change the subject, so I hid behind the cocktail menu. Two blokes sitting at the next table had been giving us looks all night long, and now the one opposite me noticed the glazed look on my face and tears brimming in my eyes despite myself.

He asked if I was OK while his mate drew Samantha into a conversation about the Agent Provocateur party they were going to later.

We sat and talked for a while – he was in some reality TV show and Sam had recognised him, but I didn't let on – and he also mentioned he was training as a life coach. I felt comfortable confessing to him why I was feeling so betrayed and down, and his attention made me feel slightly better. When I had calmed down somewhat I made my excuses, knocked back my drink and left.

I was so happy at least some of the time last year, trying to forget Pinocchio, and now I find out what was going on behind my back and it's enough to drive anyone crazy. Who knows what he and Sam were saying about me, too. Or not saying. To think that she even knew about his new girlfriend, who, what a comfort, 'isn't as pretty as you'.

Why is it that although men can make us girls feel like shit, there's nothing like being betrayed by a girlfriend. That really twists the knife.

Thursday 29th December

After a few days of being spoiled rotten by Mum I'm feeling a little better, actually. I went to a spiritual healer that a friend of Mum's recommended, to try and get some guidance on my emotional situation and my not-quite mended heart.

I only saw her for an hour; I just haven't been able to shift this feeling of helplessness that crept over me after splitting with Pinocchio, and Sam just brought it crashing back. What if I really fell in love with someone else? How would I know if I could trust them? I'd known Pinocchio for six years before we started dating, and he was one of my friends. If I couldn't trust him and Sam, who could I trust?

Maybe 'spiritual healer' is the wrong phrase – what the woman did for me was more like guidance, not some kind of shamanistic ritual. Before I saw her I could barely mention

Pinocchio's name without bursting into tears, but she cut me short and told me I hadn't been helpless. I needed to take my power back and acknowledge that I'd chosen to stay with him, even when I was beginning to feel something was wrong. I mean, why else would I have been checking his text messages?

When she said that I remembered that when I was with Pinocchio I had had lots of very intense dreams about his ex-girlfriend – the one he was still in love with all along – and I'd wake up tearful and confused, with the feeling I'd been betrayed. My instincts were all there, but I'd ignored them.

What she told me was impossibly simple, but it sliced through the helplessness: 'Yes, you are powerless about other people's decisions to lie to you, but you can still trust your instincts and follow them. If you ignore your true feelings and the messages your subconscious is trying to send to you, you are basically cheating yourself and this, the feeling of letting yourself down, is what made you depressed.'

So I didn't need to be so scared about new relationships because if I listened to my gut feelings I'd be right, most of the time, and they'd protect me. Seems like I might be in control after all.

I had a nice text from Chubby asking me how my Christmas was and saying he hoped he'd see me in the New Year. That helped. I still wonder about the Pilot, but I'm finally feeling like the worst of my obsessive thoughts about Pinocchio are being laid to rest, despite Samantha.

Saturday 31st December

How have I wasted my time? Let me count the ways.

I didn't need to spend two years in love with my German teacher's son at seventeen, when he only fooled around with me once before dumping me for a fifteen year old. (He called me later in a panic because someone thought they had seen me pushing a pram – we hadn't even had sex.)

At eighteen I didn't need to leave home to live with an uneducated Cockney boy who paid more attention to his PlayStation than his laundry, and who once shoved me in the direction of a hot chip pan before punching me in the stomach.

I didn't need to spend six months with a semi-geriatric when I was twenty-one, who made me feel fat, never said he loved me and was up chanting his Buddhist nonsense at six a. m. every day. (And I say nonsense because he only ever chanted to get material goods, and I'm not sure that's supposed to be the point.)

Aged twenty-two I didn't need to sleep with a pseudo-lawyer who poured me so much 'plonk' that I couldn't stop him fucking me without a condom.

At twenty-three I didn't need to hang my heart on a guy who was married to his job and nearly too shy to let me share his mattress. Although he was the first guy to ever make me come with his fingers alone.

I didn't need to waste those nights chasing a terribly arrogant Swedish boy with a small cock who then tried to put it in me without my consent.

Last year I didn't need to spend two afternoons taking up the new trousers I'd picked out with Pinocchio so they'd fit his short legs, and worrying over every stitch.

Enough time's been wasted, I reckon.

I'm about to go out to party and see in 2006, but I'll just type out my New Year's resolutions, in case that makes them stick better:

1. To take my time getting to know someone before launching into a relationship with them, or having sex.

2. To stay true to myself and get my priorities straight. As soon as I get into these relationships I start running around after these men, throwing myself into things and leaving my real self behind in my desperation to please. I neglect my evening course and my CV and my own needs, and in the end it just bites me in the ass.

3. Not to get drunk and regret what happens. Most of my regrets have involved heinous amounts of booze, after all. I behave outrageously: dance on tables, steal champagne glasses, pull random strangers, drink any old drink left standing around. It's not pretty.

4. Get a new job, so I don't spend the rest of my life eating biscuits in the stationery cupboard and wishing my boss would go out so I can have a wank.

Monday 2nd January

I finally managed to get hold of Samantha on the phone to wish her a happy New Year and to clear the air between us.

I'd dragged myself out to my old school friend Judy's New Year's party, and had quite a good time despite not drinking – at least I could drive myself home and woke up without a hangover!

Nothing prepared me for what Sam was about to tell me about her New Year's Eve, however.

'I stayed in and had some champagne with my friend Milly,' was all she said at first. Remembering some nightmare I had about Samantha making merry with Pinocchio a few nights earlier and remembering my talk with the spiritual healer about gut instincts, I probed deeper. 'How come you didn't pick up your phone, then, when I rang you?' I asked.

'Actually, I need to tell you something,' she started saying and my blood ran cold.

'I went to Spain, and Milly came too. We stayed in Pinocchio's flat with him and his new girlfriend, and some other people,' she continued. If Sam had just punched me twice in the stomach at this point I don't think it would have hurt any more.

I couldn't believe it. I just hung up on her, numb.

'You two liars deserve each other,' I texted her later. She insisted I apologise. I ignored her. That's that, then, I suppose.

Saturday 14th January

I've been back in London for over a week, and now the seven dwarves are trying to date me, and I think I like it. Well, not seven – that's a bit of an exaggeration, but two's a coincidence, isn't it?

Number one I'll call Rugby Boy. I met him via an internet dating site before Christmas, and we had a great time on our first evening out. We've read all the same books, like the same nerdy TV programmes and I even found out he has his own karaoke machine. He works with kids, is from a good family, cute, sporty (hence 'Rugby Boy'), healthy, has travelled a lot, doesn't smoke, likes his parents (who bought him a house) . . . tick, tick, tick. He got my sense of humour the way no one has since Pinocchio, and has gorgeous eyes and muscly arms which I was eyeing as we ate. It was nice that he paid for dinner, and he shared his food. However, he's an inch shorter than me.

I'd joked by email that I'd have to wear flats, and he joked he'd wear platforms, and when he jumped off his bar stool to greet me I wished he had, but five minutes of chat and I'd forgotten all about it. Five hours later we parted with a hug and a peck on the cheek, but I was buzzing and he called me as soon as he could. We've met up again for a repeat, and I wore heels to check if I would feel awkward. I did, a bit, but he carries himself so confidently and he's built like a baby rhino, plus *he* didn't seem to have any problems walking down the street with a six-foot woman in green suede boots.

He's invited me to his place for Sunday lunch and a turn on the karaoke machine. I'm curious to see what will happen. I'm still not drinking much so I'm enjoying just getting to know him, and intrigued to see where this leads.

Number two is my shoulder to cry on – the Reality TV guy I met in the bar when Sam dropped the bombshell that she was still friends with Pinocchio. In between my rants about my ex-best friend and my ex-ex, we'd discovered that we know some of the same people and he happened to mention that he wanted to get back in touch with a mutual acquaintance. A few days later I told this mutual friend, and a very short time later Mr Reality TV rang me. He must have got my number from the friend.

And since then? Well, we've had drinks a couple of times and I'm still trying to figure out what he wants, although calling me 'darling' and getting touchy-feely is a giveaway. I'm a little embarrassed about crying to a perfect stranger, but I can't turn back the clock. Nothing like a female in distress, obviously!

Tuesday 17th January

Multi-dating means not having to choose, so why does it sometimes feel like I'm the judge of one big dating contest? Who's going to deliver the perfect date and who's going to slip up? The more I date, the fewer rules and 'must haves' I think there are, but sometimes something happens and I just think, 'No – that's not the way it's done.'

Sunday lunch at Rugby Boy's house out in the sticks was perfect. And yes, house. Not flat. A fully fledged, detatched four-bedroom house with garden, garage and sportscar outside. As we rounded the corner into the brand new Wisteria-Lane style cul-de-sac and he pointed it out, I heard my inner gold-digger alarm go off. I've only just met him and he's beginning to grow on me, but now how do I distinguish whether I like him for his personality or his pad? And we had an even better time together than the last two dates.

I was a little overwhelmed by the living room with the brand new leather sofas that still smelt of Habitat, the fireplace, the row of DVDs and books I loved, the piano which he played so well I thought he'd slipped on a CD while I was out of the room, and the smell of the beautifully cooked roast.

Over dinner and the special bottle of wine I'd brought, we touched briefly on the subject of his ex (four years ago, yes!) who went to Africa to do charity work and got charitable with a bloke she met there, and he listened to some of my recent poetry, even though it wasn't in English and I wonder how much he understood.

We had a little karaoke session – he sang U2's 'With or Without You' and nearly made me cry remembering a friend who loved it, and who later contracted HIV, then we did a duet of 'Dream' and he told me he loved my voice, even though it was a little hoarse – and then he disappeared into the kitchen to sort something out and I sat down to tinkle with the piano keys. He re-emerged and came up behind me, asking sweetly for a kiss. Even writing about this a few days later I can feel myself getting turned on because it was such a lovely moment and I wanted him closer to me.

He sat down on the piano bench next to me and we kissed and hugged, then he stroked my shoulders and pulled me close.

He has kissing just right: not too hard, not too soft, not too wet, not boring, sucking, licking, nibbling me . . . perfect. We were both oddly relieved after that kiss and I felt giddy and happy.

We snuggled up on the sofa to watch *The Wedding Crashers* on his new flat-screen TV, but he'd seen it before and I was distracted by the wine (I know I said I wouldn't drink, but I had one glass), so I couldn't tell you the plot. My head lay on his lap, him gazing down with his cute blue eyes, blond hair flopping over his forehead, his hand stroking my shoulder, my arms, slipping down my top until he was fondling my nipple, me turned on, my head debating with my pussy. Should I jump on him then and there on the leather sofa? Let myself be dragged up to his bedroom for a good seeing-to?

I remembered my resolutions and took his hand out of my cleavage. He was a gent, dropping me off at the station in his snazzy car in time to catch the last train out of beyond-zone-six-ville. More kissing and I caught that misty look in his eyes. Since then it's been texts and calls several times a day.

Contrast to Mr Reality TV. A miscommunication meant we stood each other up the other week, and he called to apologise, saying he'd make it up to me and would I have dinner with him. On the day of the date I still hadn't heard from him at four-thirty, so I texted to give him the name of a restaurant and a time.

We both got there on time and sat down to some starters and a glass of wine for me, but the vegetarian options were limited so he wanted to go elsewhere. As he hadn't had anything and the starters were free, I just paid for my wine.

The place he chose as an alternative was fairly pricey. The waiter recognised him, which was funny, and then hung around eavesdropping, making me feel self-conscious about talking to Mr Reality TV. The waiter did, however, recommend me the swordfish, which was great, and I had an orange juice while Mr Reality TV had water, quiche and some chips. There was no cosy flirtation like I had with Rugby Boy, and the only time the date seemed to be turning into a 'Date' was when he complimented me on my sexy ears and reached over to touch one.

The bill came and I put down my card to pay for half, although because he'd suggested the date and the restaurant I'd thought he would pick up the tab. He knows I have a shitty job and don't earn much – I usually offer to go Dutch but my dates usually brush my card aside and tell me not to be silly.

Mr Reality TV seemed a little put-out too, because his half of the meal had cost less than mine. If this had happened with Rugby Boy would I still have been rushing off to the loo to answer *his* texts? Would paying for my swordfish have caused me to take a rosier view of the fact that Mr Reality TV had spent the whole evening advising me like an older friend or uncle? I appreciate friendships like that   I have an older male platonic mate called Alexander whom I adore – but not relationships. We parted with a hug and a kiss on the cheek, and I didn't feel the least bit sexually frustrated when I got home, nor when I just typed this.

I'm glad I met him but my heart is definitely beating towards my Rugby Boy and his plans for the leather sofas.

Sunday 22nd January

Last night with Rugby Boy took an uncomfortable turn. So much so that I panicked and started thinking of awful, crazy scenarios and the fact that it was after midnight and I was miles from any public transport, and the doors of his house were locked.

So, the guy's a rugby player. He asked me to stay over, and he got drunk, big-time drunk. And I got scared all of a sudden, and started asking if I could sleep in the spare room. He insisted that I should share his bed with him, and he just wanted a cuddle, and I felt myself slipping into what felt like a panic attack.

The only other time I fell asleep next to a man with a hard-on (apart from the Sailor), I woke to find the sod fingering me in the middle of the night. There was blood on the sheet, and I was sore – I was only eighteen at the time. He was my violent first boyfriend. If I'd known any better I would have dumped him.

I remembered how manipulated I'd felt when another ex seduced me on a trip to Scotland, when I'd had no plans to even stay in his hotel and I'd gone to sleep fully dressed. And yet in the morning he had me anyway, because I got horny . . .

I bolted into the spare room, sat down on the bed and began to cry. There was no lock on the door so I retreated into the en-suite bathroom and locked myself in, then texted a few friends because I hadn't told anyone where I'd be that night, then I washed my face, let myself out and climbed under the duvet. I wedged the hoover under the door handle.

In the morning my alarm woke me up and I went downstairs to the kitchen where he kissed me hello as if nothing had happened. Which I suppose it hadn't, for him. There was a slightly awkward silence, with him whistling, and me feeling in the pit of my stomach that things had taken a wrong turn, and that maybe we'd never get over it, and what a shame that was. He brought me a pile of toast and settled me in the living room in front of the breakfast telly, and as we sat and munched I explained how I'd felt the night before.

He took it well; at least, I think he understood, but it also seems that for him, drinking till you pass out is just what you do if you're a Rugby Boy. And your mates do it too. He said the worst they ever did was get naked, and usually they just fell asleep. And yeah, I can't talk when it comes to booze, but I don't think I'd scare anyone by dancing on the tables. I mentioned that the only time I'd cheated on boyfriends was when a lot of alcohol was involved, and he looked somewhat alarmed. He also confessed that he's from a rather sheltered background, and I suppose he doesn't spend enough time with women to consider the safety issues we have to think about all the time.

I'm glad I asserted myself though, and there were no regrets about my night in the spare room, even if the morning roll on the couch with him left me craving a fuck. Resolution number one: take time to get to know these boys. It will pay off. And he's promised me he won't touch a drop next time I come to stay.

Saturday 28th January

Chubby Boy never really gave up texting, but we haven't had much of a chance for phone sex till today. He wants me to go with him to a party in Birmingham that he reckons will be good for my career. I dunno. Have to think about it. Plus my doctor has booked me in for a long-overdue op on my dodgy knee around about the same date, which could kill the party spirit.

Saturday 4th February

What was I saying about taking my time? Rugby Boy was sober when he picked me up at the station, and sober all night, but it took about fifteen minutes from closing the front door to us both being naked in front of the fire, and me going down on him with a mouthful of the sparkling Chardonnay he'd just poured me. I can't say I was wholly the innocent party in this matter.

He liked the wine on his dick, and I was glad I'd thought of it because there was something funky going on down there, which disappointed me a little because I'd carefully washed myself in preparation, and it didn't seem that he had. The rest was good: he licked me out and put a finger inside me, the way I like it, till I was so wet and horny I couldn't wait, but I caught an expression on his face that made me realise he was thinking about not bothering with a condom, and I must have looked horrified. Disappointment number two.

His cock was a nice size for someone so short – hah! It felt amazing inside me too. I loved his weight on me as he's so fit, and he can keep going for ages. I orgasmed when he was fucking me from behind, letting rip because I knew that for once there were no neighbours or flatmates lurking behind the walls.

He pulled out and I stroked his cock and sucked his balls till he came, which surprised him as he'd said he usually took ages and might not be able to come at all. I felt like the queen of hand jobs. Afterwards we lolled around and joked together. In the morning we were up at seven having a fresh shag, and then it took me ages to get home on the train and bus.

Now I'm half-watching the telly, half-blogging and feeling too tired to prepare for that job interview, wondering why I feel a little bit empty. I think it happened too fast. I like him, but does he think I'm his girlfriend now? Do I want that? No. I can't see myself sitting around in his lovely house waiting for him to roll home drunk as a lord twice a week – why can't he just drink in moderation, rather than all or nothing? But I don't have to be in love with him if I am still keeping my options open until someone proposes and I accept, so why am I feeling disappointed?

I think I might still be scared to let go and love someone. We aren't meeting up tomorrow, even though we planned it, and it feels like a relief because I want to sort my head out, and now I just want to run a mile. Fickle or shit scared?

I have met a truly amazing guy. He's easily my intellectual supe-
rior, very educated, interesting and eloquent, sexy, confident
and yet sensitive. He's aware of my multi-dating lifestyle and
seems to find it a turn on, and I've found myself confessing
quite a few secrets and innermost thoughts even though we
haven't slept together yet. Not that that's not going to happen
soon, I tell you!

Another internet acquisition. I believe dating multiple
people is inherent in the whole concept of internet dating – as
soon as you log on, there are always so many possibilities, and a
score of guys who like your profile email you all at once. You
can't possibly be 'faithful' to just one after a couple of emails, so
meeting them all and getting to know them simultaneously is
the only way to go.

If five people email you, you're not really going to delete the
other four emails just because you thought the first one sounded
nice.

You're not going to turn down date three if dates one and
two were great but it's too early to tell if you'd still love either
of them when they're sixty-four. And if date four is really sexy
and makes you horny you'd do well to remember that you're
not married to date one–three and thus still free to play the
field. And if, for some reason, you wake up disappointed there's
still date five to look forward to!

This new guy had been playing email tennis with me since
before I met up with Rugby Boy; he'd been busy with his tax
return but now he had finally submitted it and was free to meet.
As I saw him waft towards me with his blond curls and pink
jumper I thought, 'You are so gay; what on earth are you doing
here?' He'd brought me a book of poetry because of something

I'd said in an email, and as we chatted over lunch in a cheap little place I know, I found myself physically drawn to him despite his sexual ambiguity, and he opened up and talked a little about soulmates and similar subjects.

I gave him some of my writing on the second date and by the end of that evening he'd invited me to go skiing with him and a group of friends, even offering to pay for lessons (the madman), although I had to say no because of course it's the same week when there's a big project to complete at work.

The thing is we're only a few dates in and I know that if he took an ex instead of me I'd feel jealous; so here I am, my emotions in a twist already, feeling guilty because I'm still seeing Rugby Boy and I want to be loyal to this new man, who I'll call Cashmere Boy after his pastel jumpers. And Cashmere Boy has told me he has no problem with me having other lovers, which, bizarrely, makes me want to do the opposite.

His job takes him away for months at a time so it's not like he could be a steady boyfriend, but I feel like writing off Rugby Boy now, even though the sex is good, the company is great and we still haven't explored the possibilities of fucking in his parents' sauna. It would be mad to hang onto him just for the sake of it, and I know he's not 'the one' – but Cashmere *could* be.

The way he writes makes me wet. He first kissed me, quite unexpectedly, over a lychee champagne cocktail at St Martin's Lane Hotel. It felt like a gay mate making a surprising move, but he couldn't keep his hands off me when we shared a coffee break (tea and hot chocolate on me) on Valentine's Day, and his touches felt heavenly in public, so imagine what they'd be like in the privacy of my room . . . He walked me back to the office afterwards and that's when we talked about the 'no guilt' business, maybe a bit prematurely but I think we both know this relationship has huge potential. Then again I always think that when I meet someone, don't I?

I'm meant to be seeing Rugby tonight but I'm still a bit tired and have a cold, and I'm seeing Cashmere tomorrow, which makes it all seem pointless. Decided not to go to Birmingham with Chubby after all.

Saturday 18th February

Would you suck my fingers if you knew where they'd been?

I spent last night with Cashmere.

Too good to write down, really. So totally different. Unbelievable. The difference between fucking and making love, then totally consuming each other in the first morning light to the dawn chorus of birds.

In the cinema he massaged and licked my hands and fingers, which seemed obscenely intimate, all the more so because I knew those hands had been wanking off Rugby Boy (yes, I did go see him on Thursday after all) less than twenty-four hours before. I gross myself out sometimes! But it's also sexy somehow, even though I was a hair's breadth away from thinking I'd 'betrayed' Cashmere, because I wouldn't mind if he'd licked out another girl somewhere in London while I was tucked up with Rugby Boy.

We didn't even have intercourse last night – I wanted to hold back a little and he understood – just spent a long time massaging each other when we got back to his flat, got naked bit by bit and then he went down on me for ages. I brought him off with my hand, but for some reason couldn't come myself, maybe because I had a bit of psychological block after all, about being with one man so soon after another. We woke up this morning, him naked and hard and me in his T-shirt, wet, sleepy and gagging for it and smiling at his face, which looks like a cheeky angel's. It was so tempting – so the best-laid plans went astray and we fucked, because I couldn't wait and I'd built up a head of steam the night before.

In a way I wish we'd taken our time, but not with real regret – only because then I could still be looking forward to it. He's off skiing tomorrow for a week so I'll just have to find some other way to pass the time and pretend I'm not counting off the days till he gets back.

Chubby phoned and we had a nice chat. He invited me up to Scotland, and I told him I'd think about it. Funny thing is, for the first time in a year I don't want any more lovers. Cashmere has opened my eyes to a whole new load of possibilities. I told Chubby that if I came it'd be as a purely platonic friend, but I don't think he believed me. I told him I was giving Rugby the boot but couldn't bring myself to tell him about Cashmere, as that seemed too special.

What does Chubby want, anyway? A dirty weekend? A deep and meaningful weekend? A long-distance phone sex relationship? Me to play Mrs Robinson to his Benjamin? I quite like him but he's so young – four years my junior, though more mature than many men ever get – and he lives in another country, for God's sake. I think I'm too busy to go and find out.

Sunday 19th February

Sexual fantasies:

- Being tied up and 'forced' to do it.
- Blindfolded and touched by several different strangers.
- Sex without a condom, him being selfish.
- Being fucked from behind, anonymously. Or turning round to find it's someone I know.

- Being able to take my time with a guy with a tireless tongue.
- Him bringing me to the brink, then entering me and shooting into me as I orgasm.
- A cock rubbing against my arsehole as someone else fucks me.
- Two guys fingering me, licking my neck, stroking me, entering me.
- Licking out a woman while being fucked from behind, he pulls my hips towards him and she presses her pussy up into my face.
- Being a man for a day.
- Waking up being gently fucked by someone I love.

Wednesday 22nd February

Dumped by text.

My turn this time. I couldn't keep Rugby Boy in suspenders any more (now there's a thought) so I told him I'd been enjoying getting to know him but felt we weren't right for each other. His reply was sweet: 'That's fine, I feel the same. And good luck with the new guy x x.' No bitter taste. I texted back to tell him he's a real catch.

Cashmere phoned from his skiing holiday and said he was missing me.

Sunday 26th February

Long night out dancing with Canada Boy and a bunch of his friends last night, ending with me in Canada's bed, wearing one of his tracksuits against the freezing draught that was whistling round the single-glazed windows. We spooned all

night without even snogging, although when I woke up I definitely got a few cheeky pokes from his morning wood. He
wasn't even awake, but kept pulling me closer. Not a bad size,
I must say, but I resisted the temptation to reach out and touch
it. I got up to make tea and we had a nice breakfast with the
morning papers before ambling over to Portobello Road to
browse the market.

Cashmere texted to say he was back just as we were going
into the cinema, and when I came out he'd already made
arrangements to see a friend. We talked briefly but got cut off
because of poor reception at his end, and he texted me later to
see if I was annoyed, saying we could meet up later. I just said
I'd had hardly any sleep in a freezing flat and was a little disappointed too, but he should have fun and I'll call him
tomorrow.

I shouldn't be this disappointed so soon, but even though it's
only been a week I feel like there's some distance between us,
and I'm desperate to bridge it. We'll see each other tomorrow
or the day after.

Monday 27th February

Drained. Long, shitty day at work. That project came back with
a Post-it saying it needed more work, and I didn't get out till
late and I had to cancel another interview I'd been hoping to
sneak off to, surreptitiously. I was snappy on the phone to poor
Cashmere, who was only trying to be sympathetic, and then I
made the mistake of opening my council tax bill and burst into
tears.

If I could just beam myself from here to Cashmere's I would,
but I think I'll stay in with some warm milk and honey and surf
a blog or two . . .

Wednesday 1st March

Sweet reunion with Cashmere in his big white bed.

Actually, we started out in the kitchen after drinks at the pub with his friends. He pushed me up on the counter and we kissed and fumbled our way into each other's clothes, then manoeuvred into his bedroom for a more comfortable set-up. I started teasing him about a book I'd found on his shelves that looked like one of the naughty novels I read as a teenager, and he told me he had some much saucier stuff, and went to fetch them from his study.

One was *Men in Love* by Nancy Friday – a collection of male sexual fantasies – and the other was an illustrated book about spanking from the Erotic Print Society which was *very* intriguing. I leafed through the pictures of girls in short skirts with bare arses being spanked and slapped, with their clits sticking up excitedly, and got really turned on. As I turned the pages of the book Cashmere slowly pushed his way inside me and fucked me till I lost the book over the side of the bed. Then he pulled out and disappeared into the bathroom, and I followed him into the shower for a quick and soapy shag.

Afterwards I found some more of the illustrated stories, about a woman who goes to a brothel to get 'serviced' but ends up being rented out like a whore to a sleazy fat man who takes her to a restaurant where she sucks him off under the table, wearing nothing but suspenders, heels and a dog lead, and the cooks stick veggies up her various holes. Then she has to drink tea made from the maid's wee and the kitchen boy's spunk. Made me laugh out loud. The second was about a naughty Victorian girl who visits her country relatives and sees the servants spank and fuck each other, then gets kidnapped by dirty, horny pirates. I think I might need a copy or two of my own.

Cashmere likes to pretend he is about to bugger me: although he says he doesn't do anal sex, the half-empty tube of KY Jelly told another story. He actually lubed us both up and kept sliding his cock around my bum hole, telling me he loved the look of turned-on horror on my face, and I was soooooo damn horny . . . He sank his cock into my pussy instead and this time I came. In the morning we went at it again, first slow and tenderly, then a bit more energetically till he came inside me. Nice way to start the day.

Friday 3rd March

Cashmere gave me a ring. And I don't mean on the phone.

We went to a Thai restaurant early in the evening and he told me about a car boot sale he'd been to in Battersea where some of the stuff was 'actually quite fun'. He handed a little box to me. I realised what it was as soon as I held it, and his awkward smile told me the rest: yes, it was a ring, but not a 'big deal' ring. It's beautiful. Some sort of Italian glass with gold dust flecked in it. I've never seen anything like it.

I've seen him every day since our welcome-home romp, and last night after the theatre he asked if I wanted to go back to his place and I said no because I have to stop being so sex dazzled at work. Plus how was I supposed to have other lovers if I saw him all the time? Heh.

Sunday 5th March

Why does it feel naughty to stray a little when Cashmere is happy about the multi-dating thing? Ah well, it's a little spice in life.

I was out at a posh club with my girlies (Cashmere doesn't do clubs – he's a bit of a snob about them) and these crazy Indian guys from the next table kept buying us cocktails. We were all dancing and this sandy-haired guy appeared from nowhere and just pulled me towards him and into step, spinning me around, picking me up . . . I felt like Baby in *Dirty Dancing*.

We got a chance to talk during a slower piece of music and I found out he was a little nerdy and a lot intelligent, and he could talk with me in several languages. We're in the same line of work, although he has his own business. Dance Boy. It got a little hot and heavy and I kissed him in a swirl of booze and beats.

He texted me this morning to say he was off skiing (does everyone in London except me go skiing?) and we promised to do more dancing when he gets back. He has a ball to go to, and wants me to go with him. Fabulous!

Thursday 9th March

Last night Cashmere and I got outrageously drunk and he referred to me as his girlfriend for the first time on the phone to his sister, his flatmate was in the room as well. Later we danced like squirrels on speed in his kitchen and then did the dirty in his study without showering the sweat off first (shock horror!). We just ate each other up, tipping everything off the sofa – his laptop, books, files – and then shagging like rabbits.

When we came back into the kitchen, we discovered that his flatmate had mysteriously (and sensitively) disappeared and we took it upstairs to carry on in Cashmere's bed. I gave him a champagne blow job to get him started again, but we were both still on a wild booze high that made everything filthier and more uninhibited than anything we'd done before. I'd never had sex with him drunk, whispering dirty, romantic things in my ear, pulling out the lube, flipping me on my stomach and teasing me by running the tip of his dick round my arsehole, till I told him to go ahead and take my anal virginity. It didn't work in the blur and fumblings – another time, slower perhaps – but I was a little shocked at myself. I've never wanted it before.

I came after he fucked my pussy for a while and he kept going, me not wanting him to stop and feeling so close to him. He really does look like an angel, even if we do the dirtiest things. I caught him by the neck and pulled him close, and asked in a low voice if he wanted me to blow him with my finger up his ass, and he asked me if I'd done it before. Once or twice . . . I didn't realise till I saw him looking both scandalised and cross-eyed with horniness that I'd just taken *his* anal virginity, although I made him come in my pussy and not my mouth.

As we dozed off we talked sleepily and happily and he even told me one of the names he wants to call his children and I liked it . . . Damn broodiness. As soon as I begin to really like a guy I start thinking about his qualities as a dad, and what our kids would look like. It must be an instinctual thing. Also, if I still hope to have a family before the age of thirty I'd better get on with finding a man who wants the same. Since I was diagnosed with PCOS (polycystic ovaries) at the age of twenty-one I've known that time is of the essence if I want to have children naturally, but it's not exactly first-date conversation . . . or even just-referred-to-me-as-his-girlfriend-for-the-first-time conversation.

Cashmere drove me to work and we got lost, because you can't argue with a man who's driving unless you're holding a map, so I was late but instead of being annoyed or bothered by his impatience, I was able to swan into the office with a fuck-off big grin on my face. Which usually happens when I wake up with Cashmere. My boss didn't notice, although what would he have said if he had? And what would I have told him? I could turn his ears pink.

Phone call from BBP earlier this evening. Talk about a blast from the past. He asked why I hadn't been in touch, and I replied, why haven't you? But that was the only stand-offish bit. We had a nice chat about the evening course and he asked, in his cryptic, roundabout way, what I was up to. I told him I was seeing someone, and he was his usual enigmatic self – he's never actually asked me out directly, too cool or too shy or both. We said we'd keep in touch and it was nice despite the awkwardness. I still think of his dick and his face and his beautiful, bulky body, but then I remember the silences and the weirdness, and I think about Cashmere instead.

Speaking of, he's going away on business for a fortnight soon, just as I was getting comfortable, although he said I could come too if I like. Brilliant idea, as it's somewhere hot and exotic!

Friday 10th March

I think I'm beyond help.

I decided to shave my muff for Cashmere this morning.

Bad idea.

I always keep it trimmed and neat – no hairs poking out the side of the thong and so on – but this time I decided to use the electric trimmer I bought ages ago and never used and do the full Monty. I'd charged up the shaver overnight ready for action on my offending pubes and after my shower I set to with a vengeance, thinking it would take no time at all and I wouldn't be late for work. Right.

I'd shaved the outer lips and started trimming the little bush on my mons and it was looking pretty smart, even if I say so myself, and it was much better than doing it with nail scissors, then disaster struck. I got carried away and moved the shaver further down and OUCH nicked my labia. Drops of blood in the bath . . . Looked like a small furry animal had tried to slit its wrists in there. Urgh. And of course I don't own such a thing as a sanitary towel.

Still, when I was done the end result would have made a Brazilian stripper proud, and the blood had stopped gushing, although of course I *was* late to work and had to make a bullshit excuse about the Underground (more like under*growth*) and then I opened up my email and there was a message from Cashmere saying he couldn't take me on the business trip after all.

And suddenly I was panicky and angry and paranoid, my neck hairs standing up on end in frustration (or perhaps to make up for my lack of pubes, who knows?) I was looking forward to those two weeks and had found some flights that weren't too expensive. I'd nearly wrangled the time off work at short notice, and it would have been a good way to either deepen our relationship or slowly, sweetly call it a day. So sensitive, so shaved, so in over my head already if I'm not careful.

I emailed Dance Boy to see what he was up to for the next two weeks. While the cat's away . . .

Saturday 11th March

Cashmere makes me cry, and I have no idea why.

Is it me or do I catch myself looking at him when we're together and wondering if he's really got his mind on the conversation, or if he's letting his thoughts drift? Maybe I'm just an attention-craving drama queen; maybe I should swallow some anti-love pills. Who knows. Something about him bringing up the possibility of the business trip then letting me down brings Pinocchio to mind, and I don't like it. Once I spent ages scouring the net for cheap flights because Pinocchio said he wanted to take me to see his brother abroad for Christmas, then it all fell through and I took him home to meet my parents, only for him to leave early and go back to London for 'work' – aka spending New Year's Eve with his ex.

It could just all be projection, but it's coming up so often that I'm wondering if I really am over Pinocchio.

When Cashmere's mobile beeps with yet another email and he turns away to check it, I think of Pinocchio and his ex and how they deceived me.

When Cashmere looks like his mind is wandering I think of the emotional loneliness I felt when, unbeknownst to me, Pinocchio was daydreaming about his ex.

When Cashmere reminds me it will be more sensible for me to stay here and recover from my knee op near my doctor than to wallow on a tropical beach with him, I think of the excuses Pinocchio made to escape to Spain with the ex.

When Cashmere says I 'won't want to go to the party. Lots of boring public school types, yada yada yada' after he invited me to said party and I've waited in on Friday night for him to confirm the address, it reminds me how Pinocchio used to get shit-faced with his no-good mates under the pretext of a 'meeting' or 'wetting the baby's head'.

Just who is it that I'm not trusting here? Me? Cashmere? Or Pinocchio?

I'm not going to play detective this time. I don't want to know.

I miss the smell of Cashmere Boy though. Right now.

Monday 13th March

I have to leave for hospital in a bit. Feeling scared and lonely. Hoping my ditsy flatmate won't forget to pick me up after the op. Cashmere didn't offer to do it, although his excuses didn't ring true: 'the congestion charge' (not in the evening) and 'it's too far away' (thirty minutes max?)

See if I care if he goes back to his 'she'll always have a special place in my heart and I'd marry her if she didn't owe so much money' ex in New York because she's won the lottery or invented a silent vibrator and paid off all her debts. Chubby's devoted, Canada Boy's my friend and there's Dance Boy for promise. I'll do very well, thank you.

Just why do I find it so difficult to stick to my own principles and not get emotionally involved when the whole world is my erotic playground? Didn't I want a guy who'd be happy to let me have other lovers? Yet what do I do at the first sign that this could be more than just fun and games – I go all loyal on him, dump Rugby Boy, *sit waiting by the phone* and can't even rope another suitor in to help me get home from the hospital.

Maybe all Cashmere's talk of souls connecting, meetings in other lives and reaching your highest spiritual potential doesn't make up for the fact that I need someone a bit more practical in my life right now. What good is it to know that I might have loved him in another life, when in this life I am about to get stranded in hospital?

Tuesday 14th March

Poor Chubby. I am such a bitch . . . My flatmate didn't forget to come and collect me when I came round from the anaesthetic, but as soon as we got home she ran off to see a mate and I was all alone with a list of instructions from the hospital which said I shouldn't be alone for at least twenty-four hours. I'm not even meant to put the kettle on. No sign of Cashmere, who knew I'd be groggy and hobbling around.

So then Chubby called and asked how I was doing and I started bawling, as though the anaesthetic had stripped my soul naked and there was just plain fear left. Bless him, he laughed at me in the sweetest way, and cheered me up with some stupid story about how he couldn't make his new coffee machine work, which got me chuckling instead. I relaxed so much that I told Chubby that I'd hoped the guy I'd been seeing would pick me up from the hospital and play nursie, and there was an audible intake of breath. Then Chubby said, 'I'm surprised you're still with him.'

He thought I'd meant Rugby Boy.

'Um no, not that one. He had to go, ages ago. Someone else.'

You could have made ice cream from my ear wax, so cold was the atmosphere emanating from my phone.

I. Am. Such. A bitch.

Chubby cut our conversation short and said he had to go, and I struggled to round things up nicely, as the poor boy had had to go out and buy more credit for his mobile in order to chat to me. But, hey, should I have lied to him? I don't want to hurt him but I'm not going to string him along either; he doesn't seem to understand that just because I'm single, i.e. unmarried, doesn't mean I'm not seeing someone.

That's probably that with Chubby. If nothing else, at least he got fit in the process after joining a gym to impress me, and he'll be ready to pick up some cute Scottish lass who doesn't want to tie him down yet.

Cashmere should be popping round later. We'll see.

Wednesday 15th March

Today's lunch for the recovering invalid is ketchup, caviar and pasta, just because. Showering was tough enough – I should film myself hopping round the bathroom and trying to keep one leg out of the water then post it on YouTube, it's that ridiculous.

Cashmere did pop round yesterday, and I decided to get over the fact that he hadn't volunteered to come and pick me up from the hospital. It turned into a long and interesting chat about 'us' and this truly deep connection we seem to have struck up in just six weeks. And to say goodbye, although it's auf wiedersehen, not adieu.

He will be gone on business for most of this year which will leave me some breathing space to, I dunno, get that new job I said I would before I got distracted by his tube of lube, and to see other boys. He said if I had any affairs he'd want me to keep him entertained with all the details. I told him I wouldn't be able to return the favour – Pinocchio ruled that vicarious thrill out for me. I guess we'll wait and see. I'm more likely to feel emotionally betrayed than physically betrayed.

He also explained a little more about not coming to pick me up from the hospital – he has a phobia of the places after his mother's death. He says that after being parcelled off to boarding school at eight he's got some serious abandonment issues, and it's because of that he doesn't make big emotional attachments. Fair enough. I feel sorry for him, but I shouldn't take it personally as, despite all that, he clearly loves my company.

So how do I hold onto this man when we're on opposite sides of the world and the ties that hold us together are lighter than a wedding ring or a promise? Entertain him like a shagadelic Scheherazade? Send him photos of my shaved pussy? Write him soppy poetry and wear that beautiful ring twenty-four hours a day?

The chat turned into oral sex, and a gentle, quiet fuck which sort of involved one of my toys until the DVD (which I'd put on to drown out the buzzing for my flatmate's benefit) conked out and I switched off the Rabbit. He was desperate to make me come which made me a little self-conscious, so I couldn't, then he came inside me and I cried a little because I was so happy, and nuzzled into the baby-blue cashmere shoulder which smells so posh-boy good.

Happy girl.

4

The Game

Saturday 18th March

The ball was fantastic! What a great way to get over Cashmere's departure.

I waited for Dance Boy at the tube station, trying not to feel too self-conscious about the bandages on my knee, and wondering whether I'd recognise him or not in the light of day without any cocktail goggles, but I needn't have worried. I wasn't disappointed when I caught sight of him limping towards me – turned out he'd injured himself skiing so we were a right pair – I felt lucky to have him on my arm, even if we were both going to have to prop each other up. He seemed shyer than I'd remembered, but he is gorgeous: fair colouring and the same mysterious eyes as the Pilot, curly hair and posh accent like Cashmere, tall like Porsche Boy.

We hobbled to the venue and I liked the atmosphere immediately. Even if the food was average and the cloakroom staff comatose, the wine was nice to slurp while we watched everyone strut their glam stuff on the dance floor.

Eventually we shuffled around together for a couple of slow rumbas before going back to our table to watch two demonstration dances by orange-skinned professionals who despite their awful fake tan were like *Dirty Dancing* and *Strictly Ballroom* rolled into one. Dance Boy is really into dancing, used to compete until a year ago, and he showed me some clips he had saved on his phone of some of his dances. OK, so that's borderline nerdiness, but the boy can really move.

I told him I hoped I wasn't cramping his style, which was false modesty because I know that without my handicap I'd be a better dancer than at least 30 per cent of the people in that room, although I haven't danced ballroom since I was at school.

He was wonderful company and we had a lot more in common than I'd imagined.

He kept looking deep into my eyes without being distracted, and I took that as a compliment.

There's definitely some chemistry, and we seem to be on a wavelength intellectually. We touched on sex a little, which made me confident that he's an open-minded sort – essential for keeping up with my multi-dating lifestyle. He speaks five languages, three of which are also mine, is about to buy a flat, and has the same star sign as all the most elusive men in my life – the ones I've always been drawn to, but have been kept from by external circumstances. Maybe not this time, fingers crossed?

I was so overwhelmed by the wine, the dancing and his eyes that I gave him a spontaneous kiss on the cheek as we sat there, and he put his arm round me and held my hand, a little limply. We snogged when we were dancing. The only weird thing is that he won't tell me his surname. Is he worried I'll Google him? Or is it embarrassing?

In the taxi home I actually asked one of his friends what it was, so I could 'track him down if I was pregnant and abandoned', which made them both burst out in embarrassed laughter. Then they refused to tell me. Boys!

How odd that my heart (and pussy) hasn't had time to cool down from Cashmere yet, and here I am having a fab time with a new man.

Tuesday 21st March

My attempt at a polyamorous lifestyle is no match for my latent co-dependency. I'm pissed off with Cashmere again. I gave him a business contact abroad and she's emailed to say she's seen him, but there's no word from him apart from a quick 'thanks' and 'I'm out in NYC with some fabulous queens' and that was days ago now.

Expectations fuck you up.

Friday 24th March

Went to look at some sofas with Dance Boy today, as you do when you've never even seen someone's flat before. Bit random. The sales people kept looking at me expectantly and asking nosy questions about how wide 'our' door was. Dance Boy asked my advice, which I gave, although I'm not going to be living with this sofa, but he ignored me and bought a horrid leather one for a grand.

We had a nice night out at a comedy evening on Wednesday, talking so much that we got shushed by our neighbours, and snogging so passionately on the sofa in the club that my head got wedged between the cushions. Stubbly, probing kisses, his slim, strong body on top of mine . . . I didn't want to take him home though – not yet – and he seemed disappointed. I could do with a guy with a little patience in my life. Also, to get into work on time for once. I've managed it nearly every day since Cashmere left, and have almost gone a week without my boss saying something sarky about 'the evening shift'.

Saturday 25th March

In a stupid shaving frenzy I removed every last hair from my poor mons, and I really don't like it. Some pussy hair is more slimming. I think *Cosmo* should do a feature on 'the right pube shape for your body type'. But I mean, where does it end?

I remember reading in my parents' *The Joy of Sex* that you shouldn't shave your pits because hair traps pheromones and your lover can bury his nose in them and get turned on. That was the seventies. Different story in the noughties. Give 'em an inch of hair and they take it all!

I was proud when I first got my underarm fluff, about a year after everyone else in my year, then they started shaving, and so did I. Then it was legs. Now I wax my moustache, pluck my eyebrows, shave my legs up to the knees, prune my bikini line, shave it all off . . .

I think we'll all end up lying in a mould of wax once a week, then have it all ripped off so we can be smooth, scentless, androgynous, anorexic porn addicts rolling around in scented massage oil on rubber sheets.

Monday 27th March

Got so bored at a party last night that I texted Chubby at two a. m., asking if he was still talking to me or not. He rang back. We chatted and flirted and he made me promise to ring him as soon as I got home. One night-bus ride later, I was in my room getting ready. *Dirty Dancing* on the DVD (hey, it worked for me sixteen years ago) to cover any noise from my vibrator, mobile charged, all clothes but my socks off. We got down to it.

He tells me to imagine I'm in a restaurant with him, and he pushes his hand up my skirt under the table, and pushes aside my silk panties and glides a finger into my pussy. I break in to tell him I've shaved it. He breathes hard and tells me I'm struggling a little because I'm embarrassed, and he keeps on fingering me while I'm trying to order from the beautiful waitress.

'I whisper to you to wait for me in the ladies, then you walk off and I watch your beautiful ass . . . '

I wait in a cubicle and he joins me. I unbutton his flies and tell him how hard he is under his suit. There's a woman peeing in the next cubicle and I reach up and put my fingers in his mouth to stop him gasping as I swirl my tongue round his cock, and we hear her come out and wash her hands as he bends me roughly over the toilet, shoving my skirt up.

He plays around a little with my clit then enters me really suddenly, making me gasp because it hurts at first, and he goes on fucking me as I bite my lip, trying not to let the woman overhear us but knowing she must hear him slapping against my arse. I reach back and fondle his balls.

'I'm licking my finger and pushing it slowly into your arsehole; I want to fuck you up the arse. I'm pushing another finger in . . . '

Fucking hell . . . He tells me he's pulling out his dick, stabbing his fingers into my pussy and then pushing his cock slowly up my arse, slowly, until he loses it and just pushes my head down and fucks me hard till I come.

I tell him I'm taking him in my mouth, sucking him, pulling back when his balls tighten, letting him come over my face, my cheek, my nose, my eyebrows, and he explodes all over

Scotland. We breathe heavily and laugh as I tell him he's covered in cum. We wrap up the conversation swiftly. I turn off the bedside light and pull my duvet up.

29 mins 47 sec reads the display on my mobile.

Sunday 2nd April

I met a woman at the party last night who I thought was just particularly tall and skinny. Then I added up her large hands, deep voice and the reference to a 'major operation' she'd just had and realised she'd been born male. I didn't ask her about it, and just found her awfully nice, if a bit shy.

She reminded me of a night a few years ago when I was on the way home from a party in a bad mood because I was being pursued by some idiot who I really fancied, but who had a girl-friend. I was drunk, lonely and cold and leaning on the bus stop, waiting in vain for the night bus.

A car drew up driven by a big, balding guy who asked if I wanted a cab. I said no, I had no money. He asked where I was going and I told him, and he said if I hopped in he'd give me a lift. I was sceptical, but too drunk and tired to care, and what's more, something told me I could trust him.

We got chatting and it turned out that he was only a minicab driver in the evening and worked in IT during the day. I couldn't tell you how it came up, but he suddenly told me he was a transsexual saving up for more cosmetic surgery. He'd had his 'bits' and his boobs done already. Under 'his' tracksuit, Victoria was wearing tights and a miniskirt, her DD breasts cunningly disguised under a baggy top. She pulled her bottoms down to show me her skirt and tights, and said I could touch her boobs – my only close encounter with silicone implants!

She said that customers would often comment on them,

'You've got breasts, mate!' Weird. She'd had her vagina constructed in Holland, and she pumped me for information on 'how girls do it' and how far to pull your knickers down when you sit on the loo. She said she had to keep a small dildo inside her at all times to stretch the new vagina, and that the hormones she was on made it bleed a little. I wasn't sure how that worked – don't you need a womb to menstruate?

She was in a relationship with a gay man who had lost interest in her sexually after the operation, which I suppose was inevitable, and so here she was, teary on the new hormones, disappointing sex life, working two jobs and with an unsupportive partner. I hoped the blokes in the IT firm didn't bully her. She was the sweetest person.

I got out of that cab full of relief that I was happy in my body, and with being female.

Monday 3rd April

Cashmere is back from South America today. He has exactly forty hours to get in touch and see me before I'm off on a work trip. I'm trying not to watch the clock.

Heard from a mutual friend that Samantha doesn't regret what happened between us, so I'm going to cut my losses and move on.

My pussy has been feeling neglected. I find myself sitting on the tube with a dull ache between my legs, like an itch that needs scratching, or the tickle before you sneeze. It was feeling so alive and so aflow that I even did a pregnancy test, just in case there had been a second immaculate conception (two thousand years since the last, but why not?)

The other day I inserted a finger deep into myself while I was in the shower to have half a wank, and when I pulled it out it was covered in white mucus which tasted of lemons. Why does semen taste so gross if women taste so nice?

Tuesday 4th April

Thinking of transsexual Victoria reminded me of a couple of gender-bending experiments I tried with my Sweet Ex, whom I dated before Pinocchio. I tried dressing him up once – he had such lovely, sensual lips that were just begging for lipstick, and thirty-one inch hips that fitted perfectly (with a little bulge up front) into my PVC skirt. We even had the same shoe size, so I could get his feet into my stretchy stiletto boots. I added a wig, a bra stuffed with tissues and a quick make-up job and even though I can't remember any role-play going on, we both got really turned on and ended up screwing on my then-flatmate's bed. It felt kinky but weird and I got covered in lipstick. The wig didn't make it. Then we realised that his feet had swelled up and gotten hot and sweaty in the boots and we couldn't get them off. I was tugging away, terrified that my flatmate would come back. He had to hobble into my room and wait for his feet to cool down so we could wrestle them off. By that stage the erotic appeal had evaporated.

Wednesday 5th April

No call from Cashmere, just a crappy, belated short email saying he was jet-lagged and had been in a meeting all day. I did tell him that if we didn't meet now, I'd be away, and then he'd be away and that'll be it till October. Did he forget or does this suit him? Am I losing him all of a sudden? Why?

Good night at a karaoke bar with Dance Boy, with lots of snogging like love-sick teenagers. I like his confidence now, and his skinniness. The only downside was that he hadn't brought any money and asked me to get the drinks, which was odd given that he must have passed plenty of cash machines on his bike ride over. We got dinner in Tescos. Maybe he spent all his cash on that sofa?

Packed and ready for work trip. No blog updates for a couple of days, unless Cashmere suddenly appears at my hotel room door, naked but for a cashmere jumper, and sweeps me off my feet.

Tuesday 11th April

Back in London. Cashmere set up a date for lunch today, but by midday I'd heard nothing from him. I called from a book shop where I was browsing to kill the time and he answered after umpteen rings, sounding groggy: a stomach upset. The conversation we had was sulky on both sides. He even sounded disappointed by his trip to a tropical country with wild parrots, blue sea and exotic food (sounds nicer than spring in London, doesn't it?) and I wondered what the hell he had to moan about and if it was anything to do with his ex in New York.

    Him: 'I'm not feeling well.'
    Me: 'Why didn't you call me?'
    Him: 'I was asleep but I'm coming into town later.'
    Me: 'I'm hungry and you won't be able to eat.'
    Him: 'When do you get out of work tomorrow?'
    Me: 'Late.'
    Him: 'Well, Victoria station's nowhere near me.'
    Me: 'Bye then.'
    Him: 'Bye.'

I snapped my phone shut and stepped out of the shop feeling unloved and rejected, straight into a freezing cold shower. Looks like April's not the right time for fishnets after all. There was no one else I could call to join me for lunch; they were all working or travelling. I texted Cashmere to offer to get the stuff he was meant to pick up in town if he felt too rotten, and then felt like an idiot.

He texted back to thank me but explained that his company wouldn't let me do that for security reasons so now it's two weeks till I see him. I shouldn't care – I've got two dates with Dance Boy lined up after all – but the trouble is I miss him. I care more than I should. I want to wake up next to him. I want to rip up the book I bought him and cry. I want to eat a chocolate bunny and chase it with Prozac and Baileys.

Glitzy, good-for-work-contacts party tonight with Dance Boy. Better cheer up and get ready to network my arse off.

Thursday 13th April

I texted Cashmere to say I could come cover to his house this evening and play nurse – chicken soup and PVC nurse's outfit on request – and got this in response: 'Sounds nice but not a good idea, busy with preparations and leaving at four a. m., let's meet on the twenty-third.' What? I looked at the book I'd bought him, all wrapped up in gold foil and resting next to tomorrow's knickers and my toothbrush, ready to go.

I tried not to cry on the bus or to think about him, but it was like trying not to think of a purple rhinoceros. You drift onto something else and there it is: purple rhinoceros. I ignored his text till after work when I cracked and sent one back: 'Whatever.'

Do you think it's unreasonable to be so hurt at being kept at arm's length? He's the one who suggested the skiing holiday, who suggested I join him on a business trip, who sent me long emails swooning about me, who mentioned 'love' and 'marriage' and 'soulmates', who told me his favourite potential baby name . . . Am I misreading something here?

He did email an apology but I told him I couldn't handle this hot then cold treatment. Then I rang my mum and nearly cried on the phone. The worst thing is, Dance Boy doesn't feel like much of a consolation after our networking party last night.

I was running late because Thames Water switched off the house supply on a whim, then switched it on, then switched it off when I'd lathered my whole head with shampoo, and then I decided to wear my new 'breast enhancers' which are silicone chicken fillets which just sort of stick on under your real boobs, only they kept slipping as I walked and making it look like I had four boobs. That's when I ended up being late even by my standards.

When I finally got to the club (with just two boobs), I found Dance Boy, who introduced me to a couple of people but didn't offer me a drink (he didn't have one either). I splurged a fiver I couldn't afford on a thimble of wine and networked my fake tits off, watching Dance getting drawn into a conversation with an Italian photographer's girlfriend. I wonder who he tells people I am? Girlfriend? Acquaintance? Person who just keeps following him around?

I had to initiate the touchy-feely with him, and there was no dancing, so we escaped the pretty dull conversation and ended up at a window, just staring at the London skyline, him nuzzling my neck and standing behind me. No more crazy snogging.

When we left he suggested we got a bite to eat and I volunteered a cheap, nice place nearby that's an insider tip. He rejected it, and the Moroccan next to it, and we turned back to Leicester Square where he steered me towards a Burger King. I was dressed up to the nines, four boobs and all, so I teased him about living like a student. He didn't like it. I felt him bristling under his woolly jumper and he removed his arm from mine, and muttered something about 'look who's talking'.

OK, so I'm not on the career fast track just now, but I will be, and he's never even seen my flat, and there I am by his side in a designer dress and heels and he's pushing a bike and unravelling his jumper.

We ended up in a kebab place where I was the glitziest thing apart from the week-old tuna salad. He counted out his share of the dinner in coins onto the table, and I paid for my own stale falafel.

Somehow, Cashmere hasn't lost all his appeal.

Saturday 15th April

A frosty date with Dance Boy. We went to a concert in a church where I happen to know that Cashmere's mother got married (purple rhinoceros, purple rhinoceros); I bought the tickets but he made no offer to go Dutch, perhaps because he was doing some kind of long-term accounting in his head about the cost of the ball. Afterwards we went to a nearby pub with friends and everyone took so long to decide what to drink that I just got something for myself, only to return to my table and Dance Boy tartly saying he'd asked for a beer and I owed him a drink. He thawed a little after he'd got himself a cider, and we had a little kiss before he pedalled off on his bicycle.

I am beginning to sense something odd here. He really does earn enough to pay his own way (and mine, if he wanted to) if his fancy company website is anything to go by. So why does every drink feel like such a big deal?

I'd re-christen him Tight Boy if I hadn't already given that moniker to the fetishist who likes to flag down women near Warren Street tube and ask them about their hosiery. He always says he's a tights designer, and the questions get more and more involved if you are foolish enough to answer: 'Do you shave?' 'Do you wear tights with no knickers?' 'Are you interested in a new design with built-in knickers?' I was so gullible that I actually waited for him to come back with his 'new design' for ten minutes before I realised I'd been had. He once bounded in on a friend when she was in the ladies' loo in a nearby pub and we reported him to the police.

Speaking of crazy people, I ended up sending Cashmere a text that would make his hypothetical bunnies shake in their furry boots, expecting to be plunged into boiling water: desperate for him to return, thought of him all night on a date, crap like that.

No reply.

Sunday 16th April

I was only away for a few days on that work trip and the plant my flatmate tells me she loves was dropping its leaves. There was dust on the kitchen floor, grease in the sink, fluff on the carpet, overflowing bins. I cleaned most of it up in five minutes, but when I mentioned this morning that she might hoover the hall carpet, she got to work immediately and the whine nearly blew my ear drums. Was she being efficient or passive-aggressive?

God knows what it'll be like when I get back from my trip to Cannes with Alexander. He goes every year to schmooze with his clients and I go along too to watch a bunch of films, top up my tan and enjoy the spectacle. Sometimes I manage to pick up some writing work for a gossip website while I'm there, although the celebrities are only a small part of the scene, and even if you don't get an invite to a premiere every night, there's a lot of fun to be had on the fringes. A swarm of photographers, translators, PAs, journalists, promotions people, focus pullers, couriers, accountants, hairdressers, models, casino staff, yacht crew, cleaners, waiters, wannabe actors, starlets and journalists descend every year to work for the film festival and network, sneak into posh parties, drink themselves stupid and sell their script/film/body/designs. I've made lots of friends among them over the years, and I want to catch up with them and find out what they've been up to. The atmosphere is crazy, part summer holiday and part fantasy land. You end up surviving on a diet of champagne and canapés, and hop from film to yacht to beach party to someone's rented apartment, making friends and alienating bouncers as you go.

It makes a nice change from ordering paper supplies and taking my boss's shirts to the dry cleaner's. This year I really, really, really can't wait to be there.

Monday 17th April

I nearly walked out on Dance Boy last night, but thank goodness I didn't in the end. We went to the cinema first and I splashed out on drinks and popcorn while he got the tickets. Afterwards I mentioned that I needed to get to a cash machine before we went to the salsa club we'd been planning to visit, but he didn't pay much attention so I left it. He bought a round and then his phone rang and he just chatted on for twenty minutes with no clue as to who had called him, throwing odd looks my way. I ended up flirting with the two dance instructors who were on hand, and biting my lip instead of asking him what it had all been about. In any case, his only comment was, 'It's your round.' When I reminded him that I didn't have any cash he looked at me weirdly, then got some more drinks.

Wine and a spin round the floor turned the conversation in a more interesting direction. He admitted to having dressed up in drag for Halloween, and liking it. I admitted to having a whip and handcuffs, both unused. Lots of giggling and neck-nibbling . . . then he said his bed was perfect for tying me up, and when I said I wasn't sure I'd like that he told me he was sure I would. A little threat that made me shiver.

He still seems so shy and proper, but what a dark horse! So yes, we went back to his flat and he put some music on while we had a chat on the sofa and then all of a sudden there was a bang and it went dark. The music went on playing. We sat there in shock and silence for a few seconds before he worked out what had happened.

The chandelier had fallen off the ceiling. The mounting had given way, and now it was hanging by a thread with bits of plaster covering the coffee table. There were cracks running out from the base like a giant spider web. We burst out laughing. Dance Boy asked, 'Are you sure you're not haunted?' And I pointed out that it was his flat, after all.

I held a torch while he clipped what was left of the wire and tried to brush up the plaster into a dustpan. Then, because the lounge was obviously home to some poltergeist, we retreated to his bedroom to chat some more. I found a book called *The Game* on his shelf which I'd heard was some sort of dating manual, and teased him about it. Although he admitted to having read it, he took it back and shoved it between the other books without going into the contents.

I was about to give up and pull my boots on when he pounced, pushing me up against the wall and kissing me until my face felt like it had been sandpapered, grabbing at my breasts and massaging them, licking my nipples, wrestling with my bra. He pulled my leg up over his hip and I melted.

He pushed me onto the bed and we pulled our tops off and we started playing, although it was a game with a dark, lusty edge. I yanked off his belt and smacked him with it, and he lay on top of me and grasped my wrists. He tied the belt round my right wrist and secured it on the wrought-iron headboard.

I bashed my head on the metal bed frame and he immediately turned all soft and comforting, cradling my head against his chest, but I'm no sissy – I wasn't hurt and I didn't want to stop. I pushed him back and licked his nipples and bit his chest. He tasted of sweat and dance when I sucked the inside of his elbow, then trailed my fingers, nail first, under the waist band of his boxers, making him gasp. Things were cool and slow, despite the passion, no rush. I tried tying his wrist, too, but he pulled free and that little show of strength sent another hot rush of moisture to my pussy.

He kissed my face and my neck, promising me he wouldn't give me love bites and lying, and we dry humped frantically, him tugging at the elastic on my pants, but teasing me by never so much as touching my muff, and pressing his erection against me.

I almost came with my free hand clasped in his, and I could feel him watching me through my closed eyelids, then I got suddenly embarrassed because this was just a dry hump and it seemed crazy to be so turned on. Then we changed angle and my orgasm curve was disrupted, so no climax.

I finally touched his cock though. I built up to it tracing my fingers round his thighs, bum and balls and never quite laying my hands on it, just sliding them in and out of his boxers. I stroked it through the material, liking what I felt. He was so wide he must have problems getting a condom on – thick and meaty, soft and not too long. I'm really looking forward to this.

Despite all this fondling, tiredness began to hit me and he was relaxing more and more as we just steadily caressed each other. His eyes were closed and I was happy, horny and not unfulfilled. He opened his eyes and asked if I wanted to stay, and I thought about it for a bit then decided to go. I hugged him goodbye and we kissed at the door, him in his boxers still, and I cycled home in the mild spring air, breathing in the scent from the cherry blossom. My knickers were sticky with my juices.

Oh, the joys of dating someone who lives close to home. Someone with the softest hands, the most mysterious eyes, that sudden lust, waiting to pounce.

Tuesday 18th April

Texts:

> *Me*: 'You left a love bite on my neck after all you liar!'
> *Dance*: 'I like to mark my women, like cattle.'
> *Me*: 'Moo!'

> *Cashmere*: 'We'll meet when I get back, on way to Italian lakes.'
> No kisses. I deleted his number to prevent drunken texting.

> *BBP*: 'In marathon. Will U sponsor me?'

> *Chubby*: 'That girl I was seeing is shagging my flat mate ☹'

Friday 21st April

Couldn't wait to leave work and swallow some dinner, change into my favourite little black number and the killer heels that look lethal but are surprisingly comfy, then paint my lashes. Not a date with one of my 'boys' but still a treat. I was meeting Alexander and his stockbroker mate for a drink so he could give me his share of the rent for our apartment in Cannes I'd booked online.

He likes to take me out for nice, civilised meals in posh places, spoil me with expensive cocktails and hear my news – the more outrageous the better. Within two minutes of arriving at the bar I had what Alexander calls a 'date rape' drink in front of me (red, berries, you can't taste the alcohol) and the conversation turned to shaving one's pubes. Cashmere had told me he preferred 'bare' women, because 'hair traps smells' and I wanted to hear the guys' expert opinions about the matter. 'I have to shave mine,' Alexander told me. 'They're black above my cock and grey like a nanny goat's beard below, so they really give my age away.'

That mental image made me laugh so hard the date rape cocktail I'd drunk was in danger of ending up on the floor via my knickers.

'This girl,' he told the stockbroker, 'is my fuck buddy without the fucking.' 'Mental fuck buddies,' I added, and toasted them. Then we took it in turns to try and make the stockbroker blush by telling him about earlier adventures in Cannes. Like the party at some villa which was seriously short on loos, and I was so desperate that I crouched in the bushes with my posh dress hiked up over my hips, fearing detection from the ex-military security guards and their fierce dogs who stalked the perimeter fence to ward off gatecrashers. Then I rejoined the party and had a conversation with Marilyn

Monroe's ex-lover without washing my hands. Or the time Samantha gave a guy a blow job on a yacht, and he climaxed to a burst of applause from the French TV crew on a neighbouring boat who'd filmed the whole episode . . .

At the end of the evening Alexander cracked open his wallet and counted out the rent money for me at the bar, with the staff giving us sly looks – easy to guess what sort of transaction they thought was going on! We all ended up collapsed in giggles as he tried to be discreet and failed. I hadn't laughed so much in ages, and felt a whole lot better about the Cashmere and Dance situation.

Saturday 22nd April

I think I should charge for my service of integrating ex-public school boys back into society. Emotionally stunted boys rehabilitated, but only at a fabulous cost to me! Dishonest, mistrusting, distasteful, disastrous and still dismissive of everyone who isn't part of their elite. Sod them.

I'm thinking fondly of my Sweet Ex, the loving, reliable, stable, sensitive and emotionally available Essex boy.

Monday 24th April

Is it a booty call if your booties are never even in the same county, let alone bed? Or just a horny wet phone call leading to a horny wet dream?

Chubby called, asking what I was wearing. 'Black trousers, green top, pink jumper . . . ' 'Underwear?' 'No bra, white cotton knickers,' and then I got bored, bid him goodnight, took off all the above-mentioned clothes and had a quick wank before falling asleep.

Maybe I should go to Scotland and see Chubby instead of going diving in Egypt this summer. Someone just set off a bomb there . . .

Wednesday 26th April

Cashmere emailed. I ignored him.

He texted. I ignored him.

Waiting for the phone call now. I will ignore it.

Don't men love a bitch?

Do you think I'm one?

Let's recap. Six weeks of crazy, passionate sex, then we parted for a short time and now he shows no enthusiasm for meeting up.

I emailed him a picture of my shaven crotch (no reply).

I texted him to say I 'ache' for him . . . (no reply).

I offer to be his naughty nurse (no, thank you).

I email asking for a call, and get a text in response. He can meet me either Saturday morning or Monday morning (and what happens the rest of the weekend?) I should call him if I want to chat (I don't, I want to see him in person), and he likes me and would like 'to know me as a friend'.

Not. Good. Enough.

Monday 1st May

I'm not sure how to handle what just happened.

I haven't had a lot of hassle from female friends about my multi-dating experiment, although they tend to be more cautious about approving of it than the guys I know. Jess thought I'd just get more hurt. Sam thought it was pretty harmless and good fun. The lady that shall be known as Barbie?

Well, I'd heard she was jealous, although there's nothing stopping her from doing her own experiments in dating. She's just been dumped by a long-distance boyfriend who's had enough of being strung along, so why is she focusing on me, and what I'm doing, and more importantly, why was she snogging Dance Boy in front of me?

Yesterday my friend Nicola held a champagne birthday brunch. I turned up at midday and started having bubbly, croissants and coffee with Canada Boy and a crowd of friends. I'd invited Dance Boy, and told him to bring a bottle – he doesn't know the birthday girl, so this would only be polite – but he didn't get there until we were all sauced. I opened the door to him in the middle of a frenetic game of 'Truth or Dare' and he hadn't brought so much as a can of beer.

During the game I'd already shown everyone my nipple, admitted that I'd fantasised about going down on a woman, and watched as a married woman told everyone her best orgasms came from a dildo, then had her husband spank me with a loose bit of skirting board, and in walked Dance Boy, not missing a beat but launching himself straight into what was now just a game of dare with gusto. It all went downhill from there.

Dance and I dry-humping and acting out a theatrical, over-the-top orgasm.

Me, Barbie and the married girl kissing each other while perched on the husband's lap.

Canada Boy lap-dancing on the birthday girl.

A sexy, sensuous dance between my friend Sue and Nicola, who fell over into a plant.

Me 'pole dancing' on the door frame, sliding slinkily to the floor and cannoning a stiletto heel in the twenty empty champagne bottles lined up for recycling with a crash.

Barbie and I snogging on Dance Boy's lap, Dance Boy looking like he'd died and cycled to three-way heaven. She was a surprisingly good kisser.

Someone dares Dance to snog Barbie for a full minute. I think this is hilarious and take lots of photos. Barbie tries to pull me into the embrace; Dance says he prefers kissing her.

Me blowing a bottle while looking at Dance.

Nicola asleep on the sofa with Canada nuzzling her crotch.

Dance and Barbie dancing, Dance making a big show of looking over at me, me defiantly taking more pictures. I could sense the sizzle of chemistry between them but I didn't know if my presence was feeding it or just holding it back. 'Truth or Dare' was over, but they kept snogging.

I started tidying up the room. The others drifted away. Nicola got up to go to bed and took Canada with her, and I got my coat and stepped out into the drizzle to my waiting bike, not knowing what to think. Dance appeared and unlocked his bike, and together we walked Barbie to the bus stop. They snogged again, and I jumped on my bike and pedalled off without a word, the rain soaking my clothes and running down my face.

Dance caught up with me at the roundabout and I shouted that I was getting wet. He touched my bum, 'I like a wet arse,' and I laughed. He followed me home and as I stood there with water pooling in my shoes, short of breath, he asked to be let in to dry off. I made him some tea while he towelled himself down. I didn't want to bring up what had happened because I couldn't afford to be jealous – we weren't a couple, after all.

'Barbie said something funny to me,' he said. 'She asked: "Are you one of Sienna's boys?"– what did she mean?' So much for loyalty . . . I really can't remember what I replied.

He stayed the night but we just slept.

In the morning he got me hot and wet, ignored the hand-cuffs I'd put out, threatened to ravish me then did fuck all. I got up and made breakfast.

I think he's as confused as I am. We kidded around a bit as we ate, and then danced a little to some songs on his mobile, me with just a dress thrown on. He pressed up against me but his dick was limp, even though we were crotch to crotch and the fabric of my dress was clinging to my bare pussy. He played me a song from *Cabaret* about marriage, twice, then kissed me firmly on the cheek and cycled off.

Tuesday 2nd May

Texted Cashmere to wish him a good trip. Pathetic, I know, and I should just be playing it cool but I suddenly got the fear and thought I should give him the benefit of the doubt. He was always honest, and he did get packed off to boarding school at the age of eight. He sent a warm reply, apologising for the fact that he could only meet up in the mornings – dinner and lunch party engagements – and I suppose I understand that things between us are a little raw. I texted to say that I can handle open relationships and long-distance affairs, but not a lack of communication and sudden indifference. Although I will keep texting, won't I?

Texted BBP because I was bored at work. He's still recovering from the marathon (he did really well), and I got so horny just thinking about him that I wondered if I should risk a sneaky wank under my desk. The coast was clear, but I decided to channel my sexual frustration energy into re-doing my CV for the twentieth time.

The Game

Sunday 7th May

Game over. *The* Game, I mean, the one I only just realised I was a player in. Now I understand what that book on Dance Boy's shelf was all about. I've been the guinea pig for the boy version of *The Rules*.

Dance was working all yesterday and I'd been soaking up the unseasonal sun in the park with Lucy. Dance and I met up for dinner and drinks – nice chat, nice food, but too much talk about Barbie for my liking. Her birthday's on the same day as a girl he fancied at school – oh, isn't that strange? We agreed to go back to mine to watch a new DVD and he put his arm round me as we walked, although he was so stiff and awkward that his hinges practically creaked.

He nipped back to the corner shop to get some beer for himself and some juice for me after I gave him a fiver (he was out of cash). Then we climbed onto my bed and I zapped the film on.

I took his hand and it lay in mine like a dead animal. *Nada*. He shifted so his hands were near my feet. I wriggled my toes, hoping for a foot rub. Nothing. I'd slipped my bra off while he was at the shops, leaving my breasts loose under my thin cotton dress. No response. He pulled his shirt off 'because it's so hot' and I trailed my nails on his back, and he stayed fixated on the film, not even making an appreciative noise. I felt self-conscious and gave up.

When the DVD stopped halfway I lay and watched him in silence for a bit, rather than going to flip the disc over for the second half of the film. His handsome face, greenish eyes, his curls, his half-naked body in bed with mine. 'Go on, turn the DVD over. I'm really getting into this film now!' he said. So I did.

When it finally ended at about two a. m., he started going on about his mobile battery running out, so I said, pointedly, 'Don't worry. You can charge it later when you get home.' And he looked surprised as the penny dropped that I didn't want him to stay. He disappeared to the bathroom, then slouched back in and drooped onto my shoulder. I asked him if he was falling asleep on me and he replied, 'If you want me to,' so I sidestepped so he almost fell over and said, 'No, not really.'

His face was still a picture of confusion. Suddenly some life breathed into him and he grasped me feverishly as if we were dancing, then threw me back down on the bed and pressed himself on top of me. That was more like it. I started giggling and pushing back against him, and suddenly it was as though someone had cut off his power supply: he stopped moving and just, well, lay on top of me like I was a mattress, hip bone pressing into my thigh, and asked me if the dress was the expensive one I'd mentioned getting for Cannes. 'Um no. This was ten quid from Primark.'

He started to tell me about a girl he'd liked at uni and how he'd stayed a night in her bed and nothing had happened.

'So she was just lying there next to you, creaming herself in frustration?'

'No,' he replied, and I could tell this thought hadn't even occurred to him. 'It was cool.'

And then, dear reader, he started asking why I hadn't let him into my flat on the first few dates, and why I'd held off so long. Was I playing *The Rules* or something?

I replied that a girl could have a lot of reasons for not rushing into sex. I didn't add that I'd been hung up on Cashmere, I'd had my period, I'd been recovering from a knee operation, wasn't sure how much I liked him, didn't want to wake up my flatmate . . .

We had a half-hearted debate about how it was possible we could dance as though we had a passionate sex life, and he admitted that when we first met he'd assumed that would happen, and there was me thinking, 'But it still might! Early days, mate.'

With him still lying, rigid, pelvis to pelvis, with me, I thought, wait a minute:

- He passionately kissed Barbie in front of me, while watching me and then pushing me away.
- He is capable of *lying on top of me* just now without anything happening. Not so much as a cocktail sausage.
- He expects to spend the night and have breakfast even though he hasn't handcuffed me to the bedstead.
- He talks about other women constantly.
- He said he didn't mind me touching him but hasn't reciprocated.

And, hell –

- I lay naked in his arms at Easter and touched his penis, but he didn't go lower than my belly button.

I pushed him off me, anger rising, and put on as steady a voice as I could muster: 'Please leave.' I looked the other way so he wouldn't see the beginning of my tears. I'm not a fucking hotel. 'What's happening?' he asked. 'Why are you getting upset?'

I couldn't hold it any more and lost it.

'I have spent *nine months* lying next to someone who was thinking about someone else the whole time. I don't need this,' I yelled, ran out of the room and locked myself in the bathroom to sob hysterically. It was three a. m. God. I hoped my flatmate didn't wake up.

I took a few deep breaths then unbolted the door, found his shoes and bag in the hallway and dumped them outside the door of the flat on the landing. In my bedroom he was pulling his shirt back on, and I seized his mobile from the floor and marched to the front door and chucked it in his shoe. 'If you don't want to be with me,' I said through my tears, 'there are a million places on this planet where you can be that aren't my bed.'

He still didn't get it. 'But I do want to be with you. I never said I was thinking of someone else.' Still bewildered, he found himself out on the landing with the door locked behind him.

The guilt rushed in to fill the space left by the anger. I unlocked the door. He had no idea what a can of worms he'd opened. There he was, sitting on the stairs, putting his shoes on. 'I'm sorry,' I said, and he got up and hugged me.

It was a lovely, generous thing of him to do, but I was tired and it was too late to solve anything – too late that night and too late in the Game. I think he understood a little better though. He also told me his last serious relationship was six years ago. *Six*? 'I keep falling for the wrong people and the wrong people fall for me,' he said, as I tried not to let my jaw drop open.

We kissed goodbye, chastely, and he left.

I composed a text which I didn't send: 'You have the social skills of a cruise missile, the tact of a tank, Scrooge's generosity and Mother Teresa's libido. Last night was the last goodbye.' Then I looked up *The Game* on the web.

I knew dimly what the book was about when I found it on his shelves, but reading the websites was like having a giant light bulb go on in my head. Everything Dance Boy did suddenly made sense – well, if it makes sense to try and score women by being rude to them and undermining their confidence.

The aim of *The Game* is to become a 'PUA' (pick-up artist) and make yourself stand out from the crowd by 'negging' women you think are too attractive for you, and therefore intriguing them so they're putty in your hands. If I turned up dressed up to the nines Dance would say, 'You could have made an effort'; if I bought myself a drink he bitched me out in front of friends; if I wanted sex he withheld it and made me feel unattractive. He also lied about his job to make himself sound more interesting – as if running your own business is somehow not cool enough and warrants the pretence of being involved in something wildly creative. And all the while this aloof act and the cold, lifeless hands.

Of course, the 'Pick-Up Artists' don't tell you what to do when the object of your desire likes chatting to you and dancing with you when you still employ a normal level of politeness, so much so that she ends up naked in your bed. If she has one hand shackled to the bedstead and is ready to be ravished, you're taking your 'negging' too far if you don't take her up on her offer. It also doesn't mention the subtle difference between trying to get into a woman's knickers, and enticing her into an actual relationship.

I think Dance may be dancing on his own for quite some time to come.

5

Absinthe for Breakfast

SUMMER 2006

Wednesday 10th May

I had a long chat with the Sailor and we decided to spontaneously spend the weekend together. Really looking forward to it – I could do with his generous company and an orgasm or two!

Thursday 11th May

I signed myself up to an HPV vaccination study today.

I had an unpleasant outbreak of genital warts caused by human papilloma virus the other year as I was splitting up from Sweet Ex. I noticed a strange change in the skin around my bottom, which looked like a small skin tag but turned out to be a wart. At that time, I didn't know that between 60 and 80 per cent of sexually active adults are infected with HPV at some stage in their lives, and that some strains (particularly 16 and 18, which aren't related to the warty ones) have been linked to cervical cancer.

Sweet Ex couldn't see anything worrying when I asked him to have a look, and neither the gynaecologist nor a bumbling med student I saw for a smear test that summer were able to come up with a diagnosis, but the skin tag refused to go away and was instead joined by a couple of mates over the next few months.

I learned it was HPV later during a routine STD check-up with, luckily or unluckily for me, a seriously sexy doctor who put his hand on my knee to comfort me when I started to cry.

I felt like a leper, and had to tell Pinocchio, whom I'd just started seeing. I looked so worried that he'd thought I was breaking up with him, but he was actually relieved when I told him it was 'just' warts and that he'd have to keep using condoms while I got treatment.

The doctor told me that if you've had warts on your hands as a child you can transfer them to your genitals or you can have an outbreak if your immune system is weakened after you caught the virus during skin-to-skin contact. In most people it lies dormant, but stress can bring it out. I could have got mine from my warty fingers as a three-year-old, from my first boyfriend at eighteen, my second at twenty-one, that mad Gucci-loafer-wearing fling who slipped himself into me, *sans* condom, when we were fooling around in a hotel swimming pool . . . It's impossible to tell, and the only thing you can do is keep your smear test appointments so your doctor notices any pre-cancerous cells – which would mean you had strain 16 or 18. It is suspected that having the warty type of HPV means you won't get the cancer-making type, which is a relief, although the stigma of having the warts in the first place is annoying. Having them frozen off is undignified too – you lie with your legs apart like a Christmas turkey while the nurse goes to work with freezing spray that feels like a blowtorch!

The other day I saw an ad asking for volunteers for this study which should lead to the introduction of a cancer vaccine, and thought I'd do my bit. I had to spend about an hour filling in forms with two very sweet nurses and to have an injection which left my arm a bit numb, but no adverse affects to the treatment today. It's a small effort for me, but the results of the study could make a massive difference to girls in the future.

Saturday 13th May

The Sailor's train is delayed. Phew. Spent the last hour frantically cleaning the flat, scratching flatmate's hair off the carpet, putting a big heap of clothes away, showering, scrubbing myself, and then slathering on body lotion. Dance Boy called and wanted to know what I was up to, so I told him about the Sailor and kept things brief. Sorry! Busy! Now waiting for my sexy sailor from Scotland . . . Off to chop some sweet potatoes and salad.

Sunday 14th May

September was a long time ago. I'd nearly forgotten the gorgeous colour of the Sailor's eyes. I sat him down with some fizz while I finished the salad and cooked the mussels and we caught up on each other's lives. He asked abruptly what had happened with Samantha, whose flat we stayed at during his last visit, and I explained without going into a rant. I asked nicely about his love life and he said he'd just been dumped by a twenty-one-year-old because of the age gap – he's thirty-seven.

After eating we went to a show and walked to one of my regular haunts for a dance. On the way I told him, 'I don't do boyfriends. I don't believe in them.'

'Do you only do husbands?'

'I've never had one of those, but in the meantime I just do lovers, friends and toy boys. I don't see the point of boyfriends.'

He didn't seem to have a problem with that, thank goodness. Once we got to the club he kept plying me with alcohol and generally making me feel wonderful. I took him to the VIP area upstairs and gave him a little private dance. Then things got intimate, with me draped across him on the sofa and him gazing deep into my eyes.

Three things I'm a bit ashamed of:

* I asked a tall blond guy at the club for his number but he wouldn't give it to me. His mate told me he was seeing someone.
* I had a drag on the Sailor's cigarette. Urgh.
* I peed in my shoe. Apparently, when you close-shave your muff and are trying to hover over the loo seat in a busy club, you're more likely to squirt your own leg, where the pee runs down into your stilettos. Do all girls with Brazilians have smelly shoes?

We got the night bus home and I got into a totally random conversation with another girl, partly inspired by the HPV vaccine study, about our cervixes and how weird it was that other people had seen my cervix more often than I had. She agreed and we laughed, and the poor Sailor looked mortified.

Back at mine we fooled around reading *Cosmo* and teasing each other for a while, then he held me and kissed me, and I felt a surge of excitement at the thought of finally having him inside me, right now, after all this time. I'd pulled off my knickers in the bathroom for a quick pre-shag wash, and when he'd pulled my top off, sucked my nipples and then reached under my skirt he called me 'Naughty', oh so slyly. I think he thought I must have gone commando all evening. I let my hands wander down to his crotch and finally got his penis in my hands. What a nice surprise that was! And he tastes wonderful, too.

I licked and sucked him, looking up into his sparkly blue eyes, then he went down on me for a while, expertly. I grabbed a vanilla-flavoured condom and rolled it onto him with my lips and the next thing I knew he'd rolled me over and was above me, pushing into me. I gasped and then just enjoyed it. His penis is a lot thicker around the middle, like a sweet potato, as it felt rather tight but good! I wanted him to bang me hard but he was almost too gentle. He came and I didn't quite, but enjoyed it nonetheless.

This morning we got up at midday and had a shower together. We soaped each other up and I slid down onto my knees, rubbing my body over him as I went and pressing his cock between my breasts before finally sucking it again, sucking and sucking till his cream hit the back of my throat. I choked a little because there was too much cum so some of it ended up back on his stomach and was washed away, then I rinsed my mouth and we laughed. He got down in front of me and pushed his face between my legs, returning the favour till I dragged the shower curtain off the rail and the water was running cold.

Back in bed we rolled around together and stroked and played but he was too exhausted for any more and I'd just realised that my flatmate had come home and had probably had to overhear everything because there hadn't been a DVD on. Remind me to buy a flat with walls made out of something other than paper when I eventually get this amazing new better-paid job. One of these days.

We went out to a new local restaurant for lunch and I tried to explain about Cashmere and my love life and nearly cried, and he wiped away my tears and listened patiently. What a guy. After we'd eaten we pottered round some antique shops and I tried on a bright scarlet jacket, which he bought for me, and then we were out of time and I had to walk him to the tube station. I started missing him the moment he disappeared through the turnstiles.

And tomorrow's Monday and I'm back at work.

Monday 15th May

Two companies have called me in for interviews! Woohoo! I nearly punched the air when I read the emails, but stopped before my boss noticed anything that could be construed as too much excitement over his plane ticket bookings. I should have just told him I couldn't wait to be off – leaving for Cannes tomorrow. Sunshine! Sea! Champagne! Can't wait.

Sunday 28th May

Something about Cannes accelerates the whole process of getting embroiled in a passionate affair. Maybe it's all the tanned flesh on the beach and the tuxedoed men at parties, an absence of inhibitions (thanks to free alcohol consumption) and of the pressure to look for anything deep and meaningful. After all, it's not like 'real life'.

Here's my recipe for a fast-food holiday romance, served on the Côte d'Azure, to the accompaniment of blue skies, golden sands, perfect 28-degree heat and presented on a bed of celebrity parties:

Day One

Meet charming American guy at lavish party. He introduces himself with his full triple-barrelled name and a handshake and proceeds to take up half the room, and together you dance like champions. Steal last bottle of free booze and hide it in a random guy's trouser pocket, then swig from bottle and share round till it's empty. Dance with guy while being filmed by his friend. Feel fabulous. Exchange numbers. Taxi home with a new girl friend, met at party, who has nowhere to stay. Listen to Alexander tease me about how the guy looks like Colonel Sanders from KFC. Decide to refer to him as 'The Colonel' from now on.

Day Two

The Colonel calls lots. Act unavailable. Despite his over-confident exterior, you are beginning to warm to him and are flattered by the attention and his persistence. His smooth American voice sweet-talks you into attending a lavish private villa party with him, but you take flatmate and a twenty-year-old male model for safety and entertainment. No taxis, so bribe random passing driver to take you to party. Arrive at villa, tell the Colonel that the model is your brother, then proceed to only talk French with Model so that the Colonel doesn't pick up on your flirting. Borrow host's wife's swimsuit and swim with Colonel, four other boys and a bowl of cherries in the pool lit by underwater lights.

Flirt like a maniac. Smoke weed with the Model and a Johnny Depp lookalike. Eat cherries. The Colonel says, 'Come back to my boat. I invite you to spend the night with me. I have six bedrooms so if you choose to be a lady you have the choice, but if you choose to be a slut, you'll know where I am.'

Laugh ass off. Relate it to Johnny Depp lookalike and Model. All get taxi home together.

Sneak into flat while the Colonel waits outside, hoping not to wake up Alexander, and take overnight stuff and bottle of Veuve Clicquot. Let Colonel take you to his yacht.

Watch the sun come up from the deck of the boat, cuddled up under his duvet and sharing shots of Absinthe. Choose to be a lady.

Day Three

Let the Colonel buy you breakfast at the local market. Act like a sickly sweet couple all the way. End up at the Chopard party later, dance like crazy people, eat lots of dessert, throw grapes at people's mouths and drink a whole bottle of wine till you're nearly too sick to walk.

Get taken in by the Colonel's compliments. Inspired, do an impromptu pole dance on a lamppost in your most expensive dress. Creep into bed on the yacht and let him join you. Get sick from the wine and only just make it to the loo in time to throw up. Let him fuck you, too drunk to care. Don't agree to anal sex, particularly as there's no lube in sight.

Wake up to his morning breath and stunning green eyes, naked, the sheets soiled, crippled with a hangover. More sex. Cheer up.

Day Four

Let the Colonel take you to dinner with an eccentric billionaire and his stunning friend (Guitar Man) whom you suddenly fancy much more than the Colonel. End up in Pierre Cardin's villa. Dance, have champagne, cocktails and some other random concoctions. Flirt with beautiful Dutch boy till the Colonel shoos him away.

Have sex in one of Pierre Cardin's bathrooms, bent over with your dress hitched up over your arse and the Colonel fucking you till he comes. Apologise to gay couple waiting in loo queue who repeatedly rub their noses. Go back to own apartment for a change. Get teased by Alexander.

Day Five
Total amnesia except for sense that (a) you're having a fantastic time, (b) you keep having to apologise for your date's behaviour.

Day Six
The Colonel goes to Playboy party, but curiously enough, does not invite you. Feel too tired to care. You have screwed him all over the yacht, overlooked by the Palais des Festivals. Cannes is beautiful and the Colonel makes you feel like a princess.

Day Seven
Go on a sailing trip with Colonel and a bunch of others (Alexander has categorically not been invited) and flirt with the Colonel's friend Guitar Man and a sunburnt Aussie. Still blissed out on champagne, but starting to get a little fed up with the Colonel, who tried to refuse to let your (male) friends join you on the boat to eat the supper you'd cooked them, and has repeatedly tried to fuck you up the arse without your consent. Plus early in the evening at the Majestic you had to stand by and watch

him flirt with the twenty-eight-year-old Russian 'producer' lady hanging on the arm of his seventy-year-old business associate.

Try to blag your way into Dolce and Gabbana party, hang out with five other boys, inherit their bottle of vodka and end up trading it for pot at the beach party. Dance till five in the morning in the sand.

Day Eight

Wake up in the Colonel's bed after two hours' sleep, still wearing contacts and make-up. Race back to your apartment as it's your last day and you have to check out. Return with suitcase a few hours later because he said you could stow it there until your flight, plus he said he was going to cook you a duck. Arrive at yacht to see nice friend of Colonel on deck. She tells you not to board because the Colonel is 'busy'. Brush past her and find Russian lady producer applying her lipstick at the kitchen table.

Colonel is half-dressed in his cabin, hurriedly flushing the loo. 'What's going on?' you demand, feeling like a cliché. 'Nothing,' he blusters, 'I was just showing Tatiana my passport.'

Riiiiight. You don't need to take your trousers off to show someone your passport photo unless it's stuck on your dick. Try to keep calm as he finishes dressing. Say, 'What do you want me to do? I didn't imagine what just happened.'

He says nothing happened but Tatiana's still hanging about. Who knows, and who cares? Wrestle suitcase out of his hand, shouting, 'I'm not stupid. I have had this in my life, I don't *need* this in my life, I don't need *you* in my life, *fuck off!*'

Escape down the pier, suitcase rattling along the planks, pursued by the Colonel. Break into a run. Colonel catches up, seizes you and forces a kiss: 'But I love you, don't do this, don't be silly. It's all in your head, blah blah . . .' Finally tug free and find Alexander who treats you to an expensive lunch and lets you moan about your taste in men. Endure Alexander's jibes about the Colonel; ignore repeated buzzing of phone. Get really drunk and return to England, drinking Veuve Clicquot in the airport on the way.

On return, text the Colonel's sexy friend in Paris. Climb into your nightie with relief, knowing it's the most comfortable thing you've worn in weeks, feel a head cold and sore throat settling in and fall asleep for as many blessed hours as you can imagine.

Monday 29th May

I think I might be corporately challenged, because I just can't believe some of the questions I'm getting asked in job interviews. I'm tempted to give some brutally honest answers:

Interviewer: 'So, why do you want to work here?'

Me: 'I don't know, you pay money and I need a job? To be honest, I don't exactly have time to do in-depth research on your last decade's sales figures and Google every single senior employee whilst I am working at another company!'

Interviewer: 'Have you ever had a challenging boss before, with a difficult personality?'

Me: 'Of course, he was an arsehole who treated everyone like crap, but I developed Stockholm syndrome and bought a crystal ball to read his mind, so I learned to cope.'

Interviewer: 'With your language skills, why don't you work abroad?'

Me: 'I'm not sure, but with your boobs, maybe you should work in porn!'

Interviewer: 'So, what about your ring, are you getting married soon?'

Me: (*thinking wrong hand, Einstein*) 'I'm so sorry nobody you don't sleep with has ever given you diamonds before.'

Interviewer: 'How do you prioritise, and manage to multi-task demands from different people?'

Me: 'Depending on my mood, I have two coping strategies – either deal with the nastiest person first, so you get into the least trouble. Or, deal with the nicest person's request first, because I like them and don't give a shit if the horrible one gets himself into a frenzy.'

Interviewer: 'How are you at booking international travel?'

Me: 'Totally clueless, every time I want to go abroad, I throw myself under a train and wait to be reincarnated in a different country.'

Interviewer: 'You seem like a really enthusiastic person with a lot of energy, but how would you cope if it was a really quiet time, and there wasn't much happening?'

Me: 'I've never had much of a problem keeping myself occupied with blogging, updating MySpace, calling my friends, watching clips on YouTube or getting a good snooze on the office couch.'

Interviewer: 'What about your previous career, as a writer. Would you not want to pursue that any more?'

Me: 'Having come to the realisation that most people who work in offices probably have some kind of alternative dream they decided not to pursue for the sake of their mortgage, relationships and sanity, what I *want* isn't as relevant as what I need to get paid in order to survive.'

Interviewer: 'Where do you see yourself in five years' time?'

Me: 'In your boss's position. No, make that married with two kids and a dog, living in the country with a handsome, successful husband, writing books.'

Interviewer: 'We are interviewing a few more people but we also have a temp in that position now who would very much like the job . . . '

Me: 'So why do you waste my time and yours, time we both have to take out of our working day? At least you get paid whilst you talk to me, and I don't!'

Interviewer: 'So, you are applying as a . . . ' *Proceeds to read my CV for the next fifteen minutes while I sit there stirring my tea.*

Me: *Stabbing them repeatedly, mechanically, manically with the teaspoon.*

Interviewer: (*clutching her bleeding throat*) 'Do you have any questions for us?'

Me: 'Yes, could someone please show me the accounts department as there is a vacancy in my life for a tall, mischievous man with sparkling green eyes, whose figures ain't the only thing that's hard . . . '

Later:

An email from the Colonel. He's lonely on his yacht without me. No further apologies about the awkward situation I caught him in, or for treating my friends with such a stinkingly dismissive attitude. He thinks he's an aristocrat. In New York. He wants me to come and visit once he's back home next week and says he loves me but I'm not daft – he clearly loves himself above all others. I'm just trying to get over the whole episode without too much of an emotional scab.

He did have some good points, though, and they keep flickering through my mind. His arrogant, deep voice that made me wet just to hear it. His eyes, his rough, strong hands and probing tongue. His height and weight – a little bit heavy to be perfect, but I loved him on top of me. Dashing in his tux. Wit like a Sabatier knife. Fucking him suspended in the net in the front of the catamaran, exposed to passing boats and the sun as it rose. The next morning I found my knickers under the table in the lounge where he'd chucked them through the window a few hours before.

He had a thing for running his hands across my body in public, me in my most expensive evening dress and him stroking my nipples or crotch, making me feel cheap, embarrassed and deeply, masochistically horny.

Tuesday 30th May

So, he calls, and because something must be wrong with my head I go gooey at the sound of his raspy, arrogant American voice. Am I just attracted to red flags, like a bull?

He fucks me for the first time when I'm so drunk I've just thrown up.

He 'entertained' some other woman on his boat.

He once tried to wrestle a condom out of my hand when I put it on him.

He makes empty promises ('I won't smoke around you.' 'I

won't try fucking you up the arse again.' 'I'll cook that duck for lunch.')

On the other hand, he asks me to come to New York, picked me up and twirled me round on the dance floor, fed me and stroked me, caressed my ego, matched me for energy and craziness, entertained me with tales of his charmed life and offered me the world.

Maybe I can't resist the smell of bullshit, like a fly. Or maybe I just want to fly, high and off my head like a piece of fluff.

I wish Guitar Man would call back.

Friday 2nd June

Got the photos from Cannes back and we both look gorgeous in the sunshine. The Colonel rang on cue when my boss was out (thank God) to try and tempt me into joining him in New York and ask what I thought about DP. I thought DP stood for Dom Perignon. Apparently it's 'double penetration'. You live and learn!

'Have you tried it?'

'What, a finger up my arse?'

'No, two guys.'

Well, yes, but not like that. One of them couldn't get it up . . . I didn't mention that, but asked him in return: 'So you found an open-minded lady to play with?'

'Oh, both times I did it, it was with girlfriends.'

'OK, open-minded girlfriends. But who was the other guy?'

'A gentleman.'

'A friend?'

'When I go to Brazil I like to go "shopping".'

I caught the implication. How could a girl have an orgasm with some random who's obviously a gay Brazilian rent boy poking about in her pussy while her boyfriend fucks her arse-hole? Argh!

Obviously we are a match made in hell. Or love's young dream, if you're a shareholder in Bell Atlantic.

The Colonel shouldn't be an option, but Canada Boy is going back to Canada soon and there's only Dance Boy, who texts now and then. Mind you, Chubby just called and sounded very appealing . . .

Wednesday 7th June

Got a letter from the HPV trial people. They've discovered yet more abnormal cells on my cervix, so I need yet another colposcopy. Third in twelve months. At least they're onto the little bastards! Looks like I may have the high-risk strains of HPV anyway, which probably makes any further participation in the vaccine trial obsolete. Nice to think I've done my bit for womankind, anyhow.

Plus I had a general sexual health check-up yesterday and there's nothing to report. Thank you, oh god of sex and promiscuous people!

Thinking a little more about the Colonel's appeal to me, I'm realising that what I crave most is attention. One man simply wouldn't be able to dispense it as freely as I need it, especially if it's in that stage of a relationship where we're both 'not sure' and want to let things develop at their natural pace.

Wednesday 14th June

Time: last night. Late.
Location: bathroom.
Activity: brushing teeth.

Phone rings. I rush into my bedroom, foaming at the mouth.

'He-wooh?'

'Hello!' comes the American voice at the other end.

'I'm frushin my teef,' I say. 'Hung wuon.'

'Who is this?' he asks.

'Blust a winoute,' I reply, irritated, with foam dripping on my pyjamas, and go back to the bathroom. I put the receiver down on the loo seat and finish brushing my teeth, rinse my mouth and pick it up again.

'Hello?'

'You called me tonight,' he says.

I am confused. Didn't I just speak to him earlier? Why the tone of voice?

'I was brushing my teeth. And no, I didn't just call you earlier, we spoke earlier.'

I wander back into my room and lie down on the bed, annoyed that he's got this weird attitude. I want to watch *Lost*, for chrissakes. Isn't it enough to speak to Mr New York once a day?

'I got your number on my phone. You did call me,' he insists.

'Well, I may have done,' I say, confused but wanting to calm him down and get him off the phone. 'Are you drunk?' I ask, trying to change the subject.

'Not yet, but planning to be later.'

'What's the time there, nine o'clock?'

'Midnight.'

I laugh. 'Hang on, it can't be midnight in New York when it's eleven at night here?'

'I'm not in New York,' he sounds impatient. 'I'm in Paris.'

'In Paris?' I don't get it.

'It's me! Not the Colonel!' Oh God, it's Guitar Man. And he's so annoyed he's bellowing down the phone at me.

'You sound exactly the same!' I try to justify myself.

'No we don't!' Now I've insulted him.

At first I think this is a bad joke, and it might be the Colonel all along, winding me up. But I ask him how he is anyway.

'Not so good. My girlfriend just left me, took her bags and is out there somewhere in Paris on her own.'

So now I was intrigued. Why had he called *me* at a time like this? I had indeed called him because I was hoping to probe him about the Colonel and the Russian 'friend' who appeared on his catamaran on my last morning in Cannes.

I was also curious, because every time I saw Guitar Man he had a different Frenchwoman on his arm, and he told me there was a certain English lady he met in Cannes who he wanted to split up from her boyfriend on his upcoming visit to London. So why this big emotional outburst?

'What happened?'

'Oh, she checked all my *personal* emails and found messages from these ladies and they're just pen friends, I would never really meet them. Just conversations. I can't believe she checked my personal stuff. I've been writing to some of them since before I met her. She's out on her own. . . . she left me . . .' The words came pouring out.

'Are you worried about her?' I asked, at a bit of a loss. I hardly knew the man.

'Of course I am, I *love* her!'

I chastised him for writing to other women. 'What sort of things did these messages say? She obviously cares for you otherwise she wouldn't have reacted that way,' I said, as my last disastrous weeks with Pinocchio ran through my mind.

'Oh, they just want money, a ticket to Paris. They want to meet a man with money, they're just pen friends,' he insists and I know exactly how his now ex-girlfriend felt when she saw those messages.

'She's locked the computer now and I can't get into my email,' he wailed.

No shit, Sherlock, I think. I'm also sure he's drunk now.

'Maybe you should try to understand her,' I offer, trying to be patient.

'I've only been with her three months and in Cannes we weren't really together, but I love her, but she keeps asking when we are having a baby and if we'll get married and so on.'

I assure him I'm there and listening, but also say I'm not surprised she walked. They don't even live together, so he needs to give her some space.

I attempted another change of subject by asking about the Colonel.

'He's my friend and I love him,' says Guitar Man, cryptically. 'If he is really in love with someone he is the most romantic, chivalrous and generous guy there is.'

'But we only just met,' I chipped in, 'how can he feed me all this stuff when he barely knows me? He was rude to all my friends too,' and proceed to tell Guitar Man just how dismissive and disrespectful the Colonel was to Alexander and some of my work contacts whom we bumped into on the Croisette.

Guitar Man ummed, 'That's just him. He lives in a dream world.'

He and I talked for half an hour, into *Lost*, right up until the point when his girlfriend walked in the door. God knows what she thought, but I reminded myself that she met me and knows of my connection to the Colonel.

This morning I had a message from Guitar Man on my answer phone in French, asking me to call him. Maybe he had the wrong number?

Friday 16th June

The Colonel is calling three times a day, even if I tell him I have a meeting or can't talk all afternoon. It's beginning to get on my nerves. 'I'm lying in the sun, naked and erect,' he'll begin, or 'An ex and I had a thing for Rohypnol. We'd lie on a rug by the fire and make love for nine hours,' or 'I like to give a woman an anal orgasm.' When I said I still wasn't that keen on having anal sex with him even if I did take him up on his invitation to his friend's house in the Hamptons, he rejoined, 'We'll have to negotiate on that.' What?

Manipulative, egocentric, rude and won't stop calling. I'm afraid to pick up the phone any more.

Monday 19th June

Things I miss about having a (nice) boyfriend:

- The sex (obviously).
- Watching *The Planet's Funniest Animals* and laughing about the canned laughter and the not-so-funny animals.
- Talking about my family to someone who knows them.
- Looking at someone's face first thing in the morning and seeing the happiness in his eyes because he's woken up next to me.
- Having someone who is truly interested in my life.
- Buying him presents and surprising him.
- His smell.
- Getting drunk and knowing he'll get me home safely.
- Going on trips.

- Impressing him with my parallel-parking skills.
- Eating together.
- Looking forward to his phone calls.
- Buying stuff together (so domestic).
- Not having to explain how I like to be touched or fucked.
- Going on walks and having someone to talk to.
- Having someone who gets my sense of humour.
- Imagining what our kids would look like and liking it.

Wednesday 21st June

Carina and I got invited to a VIP football-watching do by a bunch of corporate suits I met via work, promising a champagne reception, three-course menu and a great view of the match on a large screen. They were a nice bunch of guys, but I had a really depressing conversation with one of them, who is just about to get married. He's twenty-seven and his fiancée is twenty-two (I feel old) and they've been dating for six years, which is sort of astonishing. I have to stifle a yawn, excuse me, the yawn of jealousy.

He told me he'd only proposed 'to shut her up' and couldn't wait to get away from her. Um? Before I could say anything he moaned that the wedding was costing twenty-seven grand, so I asked him, 'Mate, how much do you think your divorce is going to cost you?' I'm pretty doubtful about their chances of 'happily ever after'.

Another one of the blokes, who I'd thought was gay, turned out to be married. He'd proposed after seven weeks because 'he just knew she was the one' which was sweet. I confessed a few recent dating disasters and he told me to hang on in there, I'd meet someone decent soon. I certainly hope so.

After a lot of booze, food and cheering till we were hoarse, I rounded up the men who hadn't gone home to their wives, girlfriends or sad little beds and cried, 'Let's go to a lap dancing club!' because I'd never been to one and I thought I was in the right company for the expedition. It was, after all, a kind of stag do. Carina seemed up for it too, and so we piled into their mini bus and set off to a posh venue which has fully nude girls dancing.

There were half-naked, fit and tarty-looking girls everywhere, talking to men in suits. We got a table by the main stage and before I had blinked, the blonde girl swizzling round the pole had her top off. Behind us, a brunette with a short skirt was gyrating with her legs open so you had a direct view of her tiny white thong. The DJ announced a 'topless teaser' – an Asian girl who came up, peeled her tiny scrap of a dress off her shoulders and wiggled her nipples at us rather sweetly.

I learned a few things. Most of the girls were totally bare – waxed or shaved, all gone! You didn't put bank notes in their g-strings, but had to buy tokens for dances to hand to them, and then you could tip on top of that. These girls could do incredible things with a ten-metre pole, dancing in pairs. They didn't actually grind on the laps of the guys – apparently that only happens in sleazier venues – well, unless they really like you. There was an on-site ATM which charged £10 for every withdrawal, which added to the clinical feel of the whole place. Lots of corporate suits being relieved of their cash.

One of the men in my party led a tall brunette over to me and she took me by the hand and led me off to her 'office', a side room with leather seating round the edges, a bare lamp in the middle of the ceiling and another fully nude girl busy writhing over a man's lap.

She sat me down and asked me to open my legs, then

wiggled her top off and began dancing. None of the guys had come with me, and there I was with this strange girl who was dead set on dancing for me. Her England football knickers and thong came off, revealing a fully waxed fanny and an interestingly pierced clitoris with one of those curved metal bars running through it. I took a closer look as she danced and giggled, rubbing her nipples and tossing her hair back. She spun round and rolled her bum above my lap, threw herself back against me and looked round at me, licking her finger. Then she smiled and slapped her bum. She put one knee up on the sofa, stiffened her other leg and opened her pussy a little at me.

It wasn't very sexy and she didn't seem very into it, but I did get turned on, despite myself. When the song ended she popped her clothes back on and delivered me to my table, somewhat overwhelmed. The nice 'gay' married man grabbed her and me by the hand and led us back to the side room. He and I sat side by side as she danced for us again.

After that I lost track of the number of dances I had. The guys took turns to buy them for me and Carina. Caipirinhas kept appearing on the table . . . There was one girl who stood out, though, because I think she really was enjoying herself, or at least she was a better faker than the others. She was from Estonia, and when she danced she got closer than any of the others had, and she showered me with compliments. Her clit was huge, like nothing I'd seen before (not that one gets much of a chance in day-to-day life).

My mouth was slightly open and she danced so close that her lip caught on my lip and she slipped the tip of her tongue into my mouth. It tasted soft and sweet. I didn't notice that her tongue was pierced until my second dance with her, when I caught her nipple in my mouth and she pressed her butt into my breasts. We made out about five inches from Mr Married's face. She told us she had kissed only girls till she was nineteen. As we staggered back to our table, Mr Married said he wanted to kiss me, and after another dance he did and we ended up snogging away until a security guard stopped us – apparently you aren't allowed to kiss in the club. Distracts the punters. I felt gratified that I'd distracted at least one punter, given all those size eight girls with hairless muffs.

We got a taxi and kept on making out, but when we got to my place and he slipped my hand between his legs to feel his erection, I made a brief goodbye and jumped out. He came dashing after me, startling me, and I had to say goodbye nicely but firmly.

That's one headfuck I don't need, although it would have dealt nicely with the chronic horniness I've had since getting back from France. Sex is a bit like chocolate, in that when you don't have it you don't miss it, but have a bit and you don't want to stop. I feel guilty for flirting and kissing him . . . But yes, ladies, don't worry if your boyfriend goes to a lapdancing club. The professionals won't threaten your relationships, but the amateurs are another matter.

Wednesday 28th June

Interesting and bewildering dreams about Cashmere. How can I still miss this pompous ass when I had less than two months with him? He is, I've realised, the very model of the classic commitment-phobe, with lots of twenty-first-century creature comforts to help him out: an endless stream of sexually available single women on the internet waiting to sleep with him, a jet-setting job and enough low-budget air travel to keep him airborne if any of them asks him to settle down.

Reading trashy chick lit doesn't help with the horniness. I find myself getting wet just watching the proprietary way that men take up the arm rest on the tube, pressing tanned, taut forearms against mine, tickling me with their hair . . . I need some action, and soon.

Monday 3rd July

My mobile rang at work.

'Hi, this is Paul. I sent you an email – just wondering when you'd like to meet this week.'

'Hi Paul,' I reply flirtily, 'I thought you couldn't check your email at work. So, where would you like to meet?'

'Um, yeah,' he's gone cold. 'Wednesday is good, just come to the office.'

'The office?' I coo, wonderingly. That's a first. 'And where is your office?'

'It's G . . . (name of firm) in F . . . (the place).'

CRINGE! Paul I sent a job application to, not Paul on the internet dating site. I blush, and start stuttering in a desperate attempt to improve my employability, 'Ah, *that* Paul. Sorry, I was getting confused . . . ' and sounding like a moron instead. That interview's off to a flying start . . .

Thursday 6th July

On my way back from lunch with a bunch of girlfriends we trotted past a feminist sex shop, as you do. Three of us went in. My lesbian friend expertly studied the strap-ons. My other friend perused the porn books. I got a clitoris pump stuck on my face.

This is what happens when you try to be too clever. I knew you were supposed to test vibrators on your nose, to see if they were too feeble or too strong, so assumed that you just put the little lip-shaped rubber cup on your cheek to see what it would do to your clit. It latched on, pumped away, started to hurt my face, so then I put it on vibrate to amuse the girls. It took what felt like minutes to find the release button, by which time I had a funny little red mark on my face which stayed there all afternoon.

Friday 14th July

Chubby texted to suggest a bout of naughty SMS. Good naughty girl that I am, I immediately texted him back to tell him I was in my vest and knickers, my crotch was moist and sticky, and that he must go to the bathroom and touch himself. I asked him to lick his fingers and swirl them round his cock, imagine me on my knees, ready to be used . . .

No reply

I bet the dipstick ran out of credit.

Saturday 15th July

Chubby got back in touch and charmed me into flying up to Edinburgh in a few weeks' time for the Festival, just before I go off on my diving holiday. The Sailor will be in town too, visiting relatives, so hopefully I can fit him in for a coffee between watching the comedians at the Fringe and having rampant sessions with Chubby.

Thursday 10th August

What's the female equivalent of blue balls?

I arrived in Edinburgh on Saturday after a hell of a trip

including a penalty fare on the train, nearly missing my flight because of an uncooperative bus driver and stressing out under the weight of my accumulated luggage. I get to the apartment and Chubby and his flatmate are there, we have wine, some flirty banter and I'm just delighted to see a friendly face after that journey and finding out that my bank account is more vacant than George Bush's expression.

So we go out, get a bit drunk, snog in the street, hold hands, have some port back at his place, me with my head on his lap. Then off to bed and he brought me off beautifully with his magic fingers, and then I wanted to feel him inside me and brought out a condom, only he was a bit knackered so I climbed on top and bounced around, which wasn't quite as wild as I'd hoped. I licked and sucked him, pulling away just before he came.

The next morning he started touching me again, but insisted on just coming on my stomach, whilst stroking my nipples and looking at my body in the morning light. I touched myself and he watched and wanked. I was a bit disappointed, craving his fingers again, and I wanted him to *fuck* me as he'd promised in our phone sex sessions. I can wank on my own at home – I don't need to go to Scotland to do it. He said he'd screw me properly that night.

Except he didn't. In fact, he was rather quiet all day, and while we were watching a film he spent the whole time sending texts, even asking me to spell the odd word. And I found out from his flatmate that he's not twenty-three, as he first told me, nor has he just turned twenty-three as he also told me. He's not twenty-two either, which he told me later. He's twenty-one, the big baby.

He passed out on the sofa and I left him there and went to bed. At two a.m. I woke with a start and a scream to find him standing over me holding a corner of the duvet, and was so confused that I thought he was about to hit me, or the guy in my dream was. I had earplugs in and couldn't hear what he said, and when I took them out he just said, 'Jesus, I don't need this.' I didn't either, funnily enough.

On Monday he slept till noon, leaving me to my own devices, then finally had a chat with me in the kitchen. He confessed he was finding the situation more difficult than he'd expected because he was, in fact, in love with another girl. Finally, some answers!

I said I'd clear out but he insisted I stay until my flight the next day, but um, no thanks. I don't need the false intimacy of sharing a bed with someone who doesn't want me. I left him a note with his keys and skipped out to see the Sailor who took me to lunch and told me he wants to get engaged this year. Screw these young guys!

He asked where he should propose to me. Me? I said location didn't matter as long as he'd thought it all out properly beforehand and had a ring and other essentials, and he pressed me on why I'd turned down other proposals. It was pretty simple: they weren't serious. One of my would-be fiancés wanted me to stay in the US and offered himself up so I could get a Green Card (however, he was still technically married), one was fooling around, another only said it whilst drunk or during sex. So they don't count, I explained.

The conversation ticked on and we saw a show, had cocktails and then he took me back to his relatives' as we'd be staying with them. We were tipsy, as were his aunt and uncle, and we all had some wine and got to know each other as well as you can when you're sauced and tired.

Later, in bed he undressed me, and we kissed and fooled around though he kept me at arm's length because he had a visit from his skin complaint. I took a look. It was inches away from his actual cock, somewhere below his waistband and covered by his shorts. He touched me everywhere, slipping his fingers in me, then his tongue, complimenting me on my taste. I really wanted to him enter me and fuck me naked, rough and raw.

I unbuttoned his boxers and pulled his cock out, stroked it and licked it. He soon stopped protesting. I think he was being too careful, gent that he is. I rolled on a condom and slipped him inside me, raising my hips up to push him deep in, and he moaned and pushed all the way in, then turned me sideways and I came after a few thrusts, playing with my clit. He was still hard. 'Have you come?' I asked him. 'Yes, gallons and gallons . . . It's been so long . . . '

We were both overcome with lust and I didn't regret it at all. I hadn't touched the patch of skin even with my lips, and I've kissed others when they had cold sores on their faces (avoiding the blister, of course) and not developed any symptoms.

We cuddled up in the dark, me still dizzy from the alcohol. We were both still horny, lying there, and I started to tell him, 'I'd love it if you just turned me round, grabbed my wrists, lay on top of me and just shoved your cock in me, forcefully,' and before I could finish he seized me, held me down, yanked up my nightie and entered me with his newly hard cock without even taking his boxers off.

Finally we were both asleep, my head on his arm. Up at dawn to repack. At the airport he kissed me and held me for ages.

6

Diving for Pearls

SUMMER/AUTUMN 2006

Friday 25th August

I've been stewing a long post for the blog, trying to work out what's going on with the Sailor and all these boys and my heart.

For some reason, the night I'd woken with a scream when Chubby stood next to the bed had brought back memories of my violent first boyfriend, the Cockney one I moved to London for.

This boy literally whisked me off my feet. I had come to London to do a summer writing course just before my final exams, and met him in the street during the Notting Hill Carnival. Two hours later we were kissing and making out outside my youth hostel. He took me to dinner the next night, followed by more making out. A week later he proposed over the phone: 'I want you to be the mother of my children.' We were both eighteen.

We kept in touch with frequent letters and phone calls and visited as much as we could afford, dazzled by the romance and drama of a long-distance relationship. A year later he had bought a flat in a dingy part of South London, and I had finished school so I moved in with him.

This new closeness only emphasised the differences

between us and we began arguing more and more. He pressured me into having sex when I wasn't well. I took our clothes to the launderette every week and he complained of the washing hanging up to dry in the living room. I cooked for him when I got home from my job every day and he stopped doing housework. He pushed me when I challenged him about the washing-up. He told my friend I 'walked into his hand'. He choked me and locked me in. I was scared and planned to move out, and he became verbally abusive too.

When I went to sleep on the sofa he followed me and stared at me in the dark until I came back to the bedroom to sleep next to him. When I locked myself in the bathroom he stood on a chair and looked in the window over the door. He stopped wearing condoms. He pushed me again, knocking me onto the floor where I grazed my elbow badly, lay on top of me and forced his hand under my top, and I thought he was going to rape me.

I finally moved out and he kept ringing my friends. He had gifts for me, he said. He guessed where I was staying and where I was working. One day he waited for me outside work, sang to me in the street and followed me. He was telling me he'd had his ear pierced so he could wear the stud I'd given him, and wanted to hug me. He'd brought a bunch of flowers. This didn't work as I'd got used to him giving me flowers after he'd been abusive. Once he just dumped them on the floor in the living room. Poor flowers. I had to put them in water.

Pinocchio was just a friend until one night when we got drunk and slept together. I remember so much laughter, taking the piss out of one another, being open with one another, having fun . . . Always champagne. He loved to cook. He was funny, generous and we were dynamite in bed. Then he started talking marriage – would I move in with him? His parents loved me. Christmas at my folks', plans to visit his brother in the States . . . I started to look for a flat for us.

Then I found the photos of Pinocchio's ex in his holiday flat, the one she wasn't supposed to have visited. There was a confrontation and lots of tears, and he fed me a load of explanations and protestations of how it was all innocent, and I believed them because I was desperate to. I tried to ignore my doubts over the next few weeks, but my inner voice kept asking why and what if, and my stomach ached.

After he'd called me by her name again, I dug out Pinocchio's old phone, the one he'd used at Christmas when he was with me, at my mum's home. And there they were. Texts to the ex-girlfriend. Texts making jibes about my background, asking her if there was still hope, a text sent on Christmas Eve saying he would rather be with her than with me. Asking if she'd liked his presents. In November. I couldn't ignore it any more. We were over. I lost it and confronted him; he turned cold and nasty. The relationship only took nine months out of my life, but at the time it felt so right, the most positive, romantic, passionate relationship I could ever hope for. I was with a friend who'd known me for a number of years, who was as adventurous as me, and who also liked to cuddle up on lazy Sundays, someone I was beginning to imagine as the father to my future children. It seemed like a dream that was meant to be: tearing through the bay on his speedboat, making love on the sofa, swimming in the Mediterranean in December and sharing wild nights out together. Waking up from that dream was a horrible shock and knocked me sideways.

With the Pilot, with Cashmere, it seemed from the very beginning as though there was the fun, the closeness, the romance and then suddenly there was nothing. Why does one relationship spark and another fail? I don't know what's going to happen with the Sailor but, for all the closeness, I think we're heading in different directions, not least because we don't even live in the same county.

Sunday 10th September

Nicola texted me before I got on my flight to the Caribbean: 'Don't get hungry, don't get tired, don't spend the whole holiday reading sexy books and waiting for any of those unreliable blokes to text you. Have a break from all that. XX'

So I did.

Well, I had a break from waiting for unreliable blokes to text me. But I packed a copy of *Scarlet Magazine*, the new Jackie Collins and other beach trash, and I managed to find myself a couple of no-strings-attached toy boys instead for some uncomplicated holiday romance, only the logistics got tricky.

I was travelling with Carina, who is one of the only people I know who's actually crazier than me, so I thought it'd be good to have her as a holiday mate. We could have some adventures together, I thought, and look out for one another. It didn't quite work out that way.

Every day we met new people, but not all of the guys were young, fit and sexy. In fact most of them were fat, married and over forty, which wasn't our idea of a holiday romance.

We spent our days sightseeing and diving, but one day Carina and I were in the shop in the local five-star hotel, trying on glitzy dresses we couldn't afford, and in walked this gorgeous, tanned blond Canadian boy carrying a drill and covered with dust. He was with a mate carrying a ladder. I recognised him as someone I'd seen the night before at a bar and given a quick burst of eye contact, and we struck up a conversation. I can't tell you how sexy it was, us girls shopping like ladies who lunch and the two boys with their tools getting all hot and dusty.

I bought a hat and Carina found a dress that transformed her into Salma Hayek as the boys looked on, and she tortured her credit card while I arranged to meet the guys in the pool later. We went to the beach where I indulged in a massage at a bargain price because there was no one else about and then we sauntered back to the pool where I ordered some drinks in the name of a friendly, but fat and married American guy who'd told us to do just that the night before. His company was picking up the tab, so he could afford to be generous! Blondie and his bearded friend turned up and we started playing volleyball.

Carina joined in and we were all getting along smashingly. Then their boss showed up and invited us all over to supper in his on-site apartment. The pasta sauce was so hot it made me blush and the wine got me drunk. We played a card game called 'Rate Your Mate' which was meant to be for couples but was just ruder if you played it with friends. After dinner Blondie and I went to do the washing up, chatted and exchanged email addresses.

I went diving in the morning and in the afternoon Carina joined me for drinks with the dive crew and some of the others on the course, including Toy Boy, a teenager who was on holiday with his parents. I'd noticed him earlier, couldn't over-look his green eyes and tight little abs. It was insanely hot, and after I ordered my first rum cocktail I stripped down to my bikini and swam out to a wooden platform in the ocean and started chatting with two local girls. The boys swam out to join us and we basked in the evening sun, chilling out. My diving instructor was taking photos of me from the beach, which wasn't so flattering as I already knew he had a girlfriend in the US who was up on her starting blocks, ready to give up her career and come and join him.

A few cocktails and beers later we were back in the hotel beach bar playing pool and everyone was pissed. Toy Boy and I had been flirting, and he and the diving instructor had started teasing each other and getting rivalrous. Carina had gone back to our room to change for her dinner date with the local ladies' man, and Toy Boy and I sat in the back of the diving-school truck with the dive boat captain's girlfriend. She was sipping from of a bucket of rum cocktail and asking Toy Boy embarrassing questions, like, would he fuck her if he had the chance? She was in her forties and he'd been calling her 'mum' all day as a joke. He grinned like a fool but didn't know how to answer. She took another slug from her drink and said, 'Would you fuck Sienna?' and we both laughed, embarrassed.

The captain came and led his girlfriend off to bed and Toy Boy and I challenged some other guests to pool, watched by the diving instructor. Eventually he gave up and disappeared, and Toy Boy and I went for a swim in the pool, although we did more chatting and treading water. Almost too much chatting, making me wonder if he really wanted me or not. I knew I wanted him. The phone by the pool kept ringing, going silent, then ringing again.

We climbed out of the water and stood under the shower by the pool's edge, looking out at the ocean and the neighbouring island in the moonlight. He finally kissed me as the jets of water cascaded down over us and soon we were grabbing at each other and sucking lips. He bit a trail of kisses down my neck and pressed himself against me as we breathed and swallowed and licked drops of water from our upper lips.

I took him upstairs to my room, surprising Carina who was wrapped up in a sheet naked and watching TV. She'd showered, changed and done her make-up, but the Ladies' Man had stood her up. Shit. It was awkward.

There I was, dripping wet and turned on, with a nineteen-year-old in tow, desperate to get my rocks off, and she'd been dumped by her date. I said I'd invited Toy Boy to stay the night as his parents had gone to bed early and he didn't have a room key, and although she looked sceptical she didn't object. I told her about the phone by the hotel pool and suggested that it might have been Ladies' Man trying to contact her, and reception not picking up the phone any more to forward calls to our room. True friend and minx that I am, I suggested she go down and wait for the next ring.

She left and Toy Boy and I began kissing again, only to have her erupt through the door and catch us. She let rip, 'I can't believe you would bring him back here! I am not comfortable sharing a room with a couple, you didn't even ask me, this is a room for two people, not three . . . ' I wouldn't have tried to have sex with him while she was in the next bed but there was no point in trying to tell her that.

I stealthily grabbed a condom and a blanket and pulled Toy Boy out of the room with me.

Down in the deserted hotel restaurant there was a sofa. It was so quiet you could hear the cicadas and tree frogs outside, and the waves rushing onto the rocks under the window. We pulled our wet swimsuits off and kissed and caressed each other's cooling skin, me wanting him inside me more with each touch. He had the sort of flat stomach only very young men have, tapering down to his groin, barely any chest hair, just smooth, taut skin and sensitive brown nipples. He pushed me onto my back on the sofa and slid two fingers into me, and I curled up and leaned forward to suck his cock, stroking his bum and balls and making him shiver. Then he fucked me hard till I came, on all fours, clutching the side of the sofa and rubbing my clit slowly.

I wanted to get out before the security guard found us (although there was probably a CCTV camera filming the whole thing), so we pulled on our cold, damp costumes urgently and the condom ended up lost somewhere, making him giggle silently, and we skirted back round the pool, past the guard who had appeared and up to my room because Toy Boy still had no place to stay.

Carina was furious, and while I stood there in my cold, damp bikini with a condom wrapper wedged in the cup, and my embarrassed teenager standing sheepishly next to me, I gestured with the arm with the blanket on it and knocked over a rum bottle which smashed. Toy Boy stepped on a shard of glass and there was blood everywhere, and Carina went on ranting and shouting at me. I found a wash cloth and ran it under the tap to press it on Toy Boy's wound, and then Carina snapped to and found some plasters. She thrust our dive-instructor's number on Toy Boy, suggesting he crashed at his place. The poor boy was confused and humiliated, tired and injured with nowhere to go.

We went outside to call his parents but there was no response, and I was determined not to chuck him out on the dark street, bleeding, after I'd just ravished him. Carina poked her head out of the door, maybe having heard us, and said he could stay after all. She probably regretted it later as he barely slept, snuggled up next to me, but went on kissing and fondling me. In the morning she vanished and we fucked again, in comfort.

The next night Carina and I went out clubbing with Blondie, some of his work mates and Toy Boy, who kept a straight face when I introduced him to Blondie. Toy Boy and I had spent the day's diving getting to know each other, and were on the way to being thick as thieves. I also knew he was bi, and he whispered to me that he fancied Blondie too. He didn't let on to him that we'd been desecrating the restaurant sofa twelve hours earlier, and Blondie seemed to think Toy Boy was my new surrogate little brother. After hours of dancing I was tired and horny, desperate to be alone with Blondie. Carina had come round to Toy Boy after several cocktails, and even told him he could stay at our place as it was too late to go to the other end of the island and wake up his parents. This was great news, but I wasn't planning to stay the night in our room – I was going back with Blondie, and Toy Boy didn't mind. We were mates now, even if we'd had a one-off 'extra' – and he knew I fancied Blondie. With the karaoke blasting out behind us, I broke the news to Carina and watched her face change.

'*I cannot be responsible for your love life!*' she screamed.

'What? I didn't ask you to,' I had to yell back to make myself heard. 'It's fine, don't worry! You don't have to do anything!'

'But I offered your lover to stay in our room, and now you're going back with this other guy?! This is not my problem! Not my problem!' she was so angry that her English started to falter.

'I'm not asking you to lie for me.' I looked round anxiously to see if Blondie and his mates had heard, but they seemed to be oblivious. Obviously two screaming women were par for the course as far as they were concerned. 'Shhhh, Carina, don't scream at me. Toy Boy knows, he doesn't mind.'

'What are you going to do when Blondie finds out? I am not lying for you!'

'You don't have to, I don't want . . .'

'I am not telling stories so you can cheat on boys!'

'It's not cheating, Carina – neither of them are my boyfriend. You don't have to do anything or say anything. Honest.'

'*I cannot be responsible for your love life!*' she shouted at me again.

She seemed to think that she'd done me a favour by generously offering Toy Boy to crash in our room again, instead she had just made a huge mess of my plans. Stubborn, and frothing at the mouth with jealousy, she now refused to stay in our room with Toy Boy without me, and left on the back of some tanned boy's motorcycle.

I gave up and walked back to Blondie, hooked an arm in his and led him out of the club. There were no cabs so we walked back to the hotel where he worked in the hot, sticky dark. He had an apartment which he shared with his friend, and it was pretty filthy, with overflowing bins. I was dying for a shower, and he showed me how it worked and left me to it. The thought crossed my mind that I'd prefer to take a bubble bath with him, so I opened the taps full blast and began pouring in shampoo and shower gel. Then I turned off the light.

A few seconds later he popped his head round the door, wondering why I wasn't done yet, and I told him to climb in the bath. I all but closed the door behind him so it was nearly pitch black, pulled off my towel and hung it over the shower curtain rail, then slipped under the bubbles. I watched him strip in silhouette and climb in and sit in front of me.

He sat between my thighs and I massaged his shoulders, then grabbed more conditioner and lubricated his back and neck. He moaned with pleasure, and I could tell he was hard. My hand grazed his penis as I stroked and hugged him, but I didn't touch it yet.

Then his flatmate and Toy Boy came into the flat, obviously avoiding Carina's wrath. I bet Blondie's mate didn't need an explanation – girls, and Latin ones in particular, are a mystery to most boys anyway. We tried to keep quiet, then giggled and splashed a bit, so the others would get the message, then they turned off the bedroom lights and it really was pitch black. We were suspended in the warm water and bubbles, almost strangers. Any sound echoed back off the bathroom tiles, and the door was ajar, but I forgot to feel self-conscious after a while. Blondie's hands were wrinkly from the water and rough from work, but with the shower gel they were soft when they massaged my nipples, and his kisses were warm. The bath was wide enough for us to lie side by side and I explored his body in the dark. He was a tiny bit shorter than me, but his hands and penis were a generous size when I reached down below his waist for the first time.

I went down on him, imagining his clear blue eyes watching me under his floppy blond hair. His belly was muscled and flat, and he'd shaved his pubes. I touched and stroked his balls for a few seconds, then took his smooth penis into my mouth. He moaned and splashed and I thought about the two other boys and what would happen if they burst in on us. Two of them with hard-ons, holding me down while the third had his way with me, raw, sexy and urgent, the slip of the bathwater. Then taking on the next one . . . Unfortunately, I think they were asleep after all.

I blew Blondie, half in and half out of the water, holding my breath using the techniques I'd learned in my diving class, breathing out through my nose. He clutched me ecstatically, then slid two fingers inside me and straight onto my G-spot which felt like he was flicking a switch. I reached down and pressed my clit and came suddenly, with amazing intensity, feeling that flood deep inside me and not wanting him to ever stop being my lover.

I turned over in the bath so he could slide his cock into me and pump away for a few seconds, before pushing him away, lying back and pulling him between my legs, my head up against the bath edge, our pelvises sealed together, and he pushed himself back into me. After a few seconds, scolding myself for being so horny and stupid, I got up and out of the water.

We continued on the double sofa bed in the living room, me tugging a condom on him, and he bent over me, lifted my legs up and banged me hard and fast and without a drop of tenderness. I could finally see his gorgeous face staring at his dick as it rammed into my pussy. We collapsed together and he was asleep in seconds.

I spent the next few days skirting Carina's moods, spending my days with Toy Boy and my nights with Blondie. I didn't sleep with Toy Boy again, although we kept up the chemistry. One night we all snuck into the hotel Jacuzzi after hours and when Blondie nipped off to the loo I took the opportunity to have a quick fumble in the bubbles with my nineteen year old.

Even Carina eventually managed to chill out following regular, relaxing massage treatments on the beach and a rekindled romance with Ladies' Man, who explained his absence from their date by having fallen asleep after too much weed. We left the island with huge, satisfied grins and bulging suitcases, containing huge amounts of rum.

Tuesday 12th September

Jet lag sucks when your young, blond lover comes online from halfway round the world and then his connection is gone after thirty seconds when your bloody computer commits temporary suicide. We'd been messaging about sex in the pool, his perfect cock in me, his fingers finding my horniest spot like a precision-guided missile, sweaty walks across the golf course back to his hotel, his dirty, beautiful mouth and rough hands, his thick tongue in my mouth, kissing in the warm ocean with cold rain falling . . .

Intrigued by this whole G-spot experience, I consulted my friend Nicola, who told me it happened all the time for her. Apparently she's disappointed if she 'only' has a clitoral orgasm, and that it's easy – 'You just use men's willies to rub against it.' I wasn't totally sure how this worked, so I phoned Canada Boy, who'd slept with Nicola the night of her champagne birthday party.

'How does she do it?' I demanded, once the small talk was over and I'd explained what I was phoning about.

'She said she uses the man? What did she mean?' He sounded embarrassed and confused.

'I don't know – what did she do differently that no other girl does?'

'Well, she just sort of gyrates . . . '

Looks like I will have to ask her for a demonstration after all. The Rabbit's just not doing it for me.

Wednesday 11th October

Eighteen months ago I wouldn't have thought that I would:

- Have slept with as many people as I have.
- Have kept writing about my sex life for a year.
- Have finally gotten over Pinocchio.
- Have lost touch with so many friends.
- Have had sex with a herpes carrier.
- Have had to teach a woman in her thirties that a flat doesn't clean itself.
- Still believe every lie I hear.
- Fall for the gayest-looking straight man I'd ever clapped eyes on (Cashmere).
- Still be no nearer starting that family; I haven't even met one decent prospect.
- Have slept with someone the age of my little cousin.
- Be in a position to buy a flat myself.

And I am! I got the job – the one with the bigger salary, the one with the most chance for career progression and getting to make more decisions on a daily basis, but mostly the salary that means I can finally get my own place and not have to talk flat-mate through basics like bin emptying and hoovering.

I'd be even happier if I hadn't just logged onto my old favourite dating site and discovered that Cashmere is back in town and has been really active. Cash – 'I don't do closure' – mere. Nice.

Half of me wants to throw myself back into the multi-dating melee, half is pulling back. I'll start to muddle up these guys, and get exhausted running around with them all. I'll pick the wrong one or sleep with all of them and feel like a slut. They might find out about each other, not like it and get hurt or hurt me. Or I will fall for more than one of them at a time and not be able to choose, then be back to just me, starting all over again.

The Colonel is still emailing and I had some sweet messages from the Sailor, but I'm swallowing back the anger about Cashmere. Damn.

7

Kensington Nights

AUTUMN/WINTER 2006

Monday 16th October

Cashmere still hasn't called me. He's still busy on the dating site. I'm busy on the web too, looking up mortgage advice online, because I found a flat! It all happened so fast that I am now a serious convert to that cosmic ordering thing where you concentrate on a thought and then follow all the pathways that open to make it a reality.

I took Alexander along to the viewing for moral support – after all, he is the only person I know who actually owns properties and who was able to give me qualified advice.

I was worried I wouldn't have much of a chance when it came to making an offer, when I saw all the other would-be buyers milling around the flat, but it's everything I've dreamed of and more: new, clean, with a working cooker and non-draughty windows, much quieter than my current place and with crackless walls and proper water pressure in the shower!

I can't cope with my flatmate's mess any more, or not having a living room. I just want to have all my stuff in one place and never feel like I might have to pack everything up and move on or that I have to keep my landlord sweet or else be out on my ear. I'll have to have a rent-paying lodger too, but if it's my place

I'm sure that'll be tolerable. I really want this to happen. There's got to be a bit of stability somewhere in my life, even if it's not in my love life.

I love my new job already. It's a tiny company, just me, the boss and a bunch of freelancers who come in to work on specific projects so hopefully I can be a bit more involved with something more career-building than admin. I can wear pretty much what I want to – they're laidback about it, and it doesn't matter if I get in a bit late as long as I make it up in the evening.

Friday 20th October

When one door closes, another door opens. In my case, when a couple of men exit the revolving door, a couple more tumble in. Today one tumbled into my lap, or at least into my office. Our new graphic designer. And he's freelance but he's going to be working with us for a while so apparently I'll be seeing a lot of him. Did I mention how much I love my job?

I opened the door in a short, red dress and there he was, tall, stubbly and smiling on the doorstep, with a big file of his designs under one arm and the sun in his blue eyes. I brought him in and showed him round the office and found him the only other free desk – opposite mine – and in no time we had fallen into a groove of teasing, bantering conversation. Then my boss appeared and whisked him away to his room for a meeting, and I tried to get on with what I'd been doing before I was so divinely interrupted.

He's so tall I don't dare look at him when he's standing next to me in case I get vertigo and faint, or in case my blush gives me away. This morning I spotted a copy of *Girl with a One Track Mind* in his bag, and we had a natter about it, with some kind of flirty electrical charge sparking in the air.

He told me he was 'really enjoying it' but 'couldn't believe any girl would actually think and act like that', and I smiled my secret smile, said nothing and clicked the entry I'd been typing for my blog behind a spreadsheet.

I crashed on the office sofa at lunch with a copy of *Cosmo*, thinking I was too old to be reading articles called things like 'How to turn bad sex into good sex' (why not just stop and get a new man to shag? One who's actually good in bed?) and he sat at his desk messaging and eating a yoghurt.

He does what I do: licks the yoghurt off the foil lid. I had one eye on the magazine and one on that tongue on the foil. He was very patient and particular, as though he was enjoying himself thoroughly. I was enjoying watching, feeling dirtier by the minute, unable to concentrate on more than a paragraph of the article at a time. Why bother with bad sex when you can watch Tall Boy's tongue caressing a yoghurt pot?

Wednesday 1st November

Something outrageous happened last weekend at Lucy's boyfriend's birthday party that I still can't quite believe, making me wonder how many drinks it takes for me to find myself in a rooftop Jacuzzi, being fondled by two men and fingering another girl? To be honest, I can't remember.

Which doesn't stop me feeling a curious mix of mortal embarrassment and wicked excitement from the memory.

It was a full-blown party. There were people dancing, drinking and mingling innocently around us as we sat and bubbled away in the warm water, me with two people's hands in my crotch and my fist round a penis. Honestly, I don't know what possessed me. The evening started inconspicuously enough with some wine at a pub, followed by more wine, but as soon as I mixed myself a tumbler of vodka and orange back at my host's flat high above the roofs of London and stripped down to my corset and knickers to join the tame-looking people in the hot tub, things started getting out of hand.

Instantly, one man with a shaved head (something I loathe), pulled me towards him and started kissing me without so much as introducing himself. I tried to keep my composure and chat to two gay guys sitting next to me, and Shaved Head kept on kissing the back of my neck and stroking me under water, under cover of the bubbles. It felt nice, and I was buzzing from the alcohol and the music. I called out to another guy who wandered near enough for me to grab his arm and soak his expensive shirt, so he grinned, unbuttoned his shirt and pulled it and his trousers off and sank into the pool beside me. I called him 'Hugh' all night, which I later found out wasn't even his name – hopefully he just thought I was saying 'you' breathily.

Next thing I was kissing him and getting horny. The music, the alcohol, the warm water and the brush of random hands under the water, laughter, and wet, drooping cigarettes . . . I stood up and danced and 'Hugh' pulled me back into the pool. The atmosphere was surreal and dreamlike, then suddenly his hand tugged at the elastic of my knickers and his finger pushed into me. He began to thrust, twist and pull away his finger with an urgent, pulsing rhythm that turned me on more intensely than a mere tickle on the clit. Then he pushed a finger into my anus, which was rather uncomfortable.

I rested a hand on his cock, kissing him hard, oblivious to everyone around us. Shaved Head was on the other side of me, watching us and stroking me, grinding my knickers against my clitoris, his fist between my thighs, above my other suitor's hand. 'Hugh' wasn't getting fully hard, but he seemed to get a lot of pleasure from feeling me squirm with lust on his lap. I was so turned on I could hardly speak. 'No, don't, please, no, please don't,' was all I could say, but I meant the opposite, and was crashing towards a huge orgasm. 'Why not?' he asked, with a naughty glint in his eye. The distinct impression penetrated through my brain, turned to mush with booze, sex and warm water, that he was trying to manoeuvre me so he could fuck me or push himself into my arse.

Just when things were reaching a pitch, a guy I'd got on with well at the bar joined the mass of bodies in the Jacuzzi with a petite brunette girl and somehow the intensity cut and we were all just talking and flirting again.

Until, unexpectedly, the girl started to kiss me, slowly at first and then more urgently, pressing herself into me. She tasted like an ash tray, but her lips were soft and probing and – I can't remember if I was bold and did it or she put my hand there – I was shoving my fingers into her pants and through her muff.

Women's bodies are just so different to men's. Instead of a hard, pulsing cock there was soft wetness, curls of hair, flab, a hole . . . I poked one finger into her pussy and she moaned into my ear, grinding against me, pressing my hand deeper. For a while, I enjoyed these new sensations, but then I began to feel a bit sick from her nicotine tongue, and all the alcohol made my head swim, so I decided to call it a night. Touching her was odd, and did nothing for me after I'd satisfied my initial curiosity – like being forced to stroke a snake when you'd rather cradle a hamster (or the opposite, in this case). I climbed out of the pool and dried off on some towels the host had laid out, shivering in the November night.

'Hugh' offered to take me home but I went with the brunette's companion instead, who was a perfect gent and dropped me off on my doorstep without even complaining that the outside of his car door was covered in vomit. Nothing else happened, and I didn't want it to. I had the hangover from hell today – it's four p. m. and it's still with me, despite junk food and litres of water. Who was that girl? Was she a lesbian? She certainly insisted I would be the only person she kissed, and I only wish she'd been a non-smoker. I touched her half out of curiosity, half because she expected me to, and I didn't know how to politely refuse. And if she hadn't climbed in, would I have fucked 'Hugh' right there and then, surrounded by people who were fully dressed and watching? Totally unprotected? Probably not, but a scary thought.

Friday 3rd November

I have to say I've never fancied girls or even had 'a crush' on a teacher. A few years ago I shared a bed with a female friend and she asked me to kiss her, but the whole experience was just odd and not particularly sexy. The lap dancing club was the only time it's stirred me – that Estonian girl who smelled so amazing, who liked me, kissed me, hooked me in. My pussy slicked up as I tried to catch her nipple in my mouth. What if she'd been the one in the Jacuzzi?

Last night I had one of those erotic dreams that feel like a shock. A tall, beautiful woman with a short blonde bob, large breasts and a lithe body came close to my face, exposed her breasts, kissed me passionately and mounted me, her bare breasts in my face. Then I woke up and had an early morning wank.

It is Friday after all.

Wednesday 8th November

I wrangled Tall Boy out to the theatre tonight, without calling it a 'date'. We'd flirted back and forth on email all day, went our separate ways for supper and met in the theatre bar just before the show. The play was good, if a bit dark. 'Typical,' I remarked in the interval. 'A guy opens up emotionally and makes himself vulnerable, then he feels stupid and undignified and leaves the woman, never to be heard from again.' Exactly what happened with Cashmere. 'The woman, meanwhile, would be happy to love the man, warts, emotional scars and all, but he disappears in a puff of smoke . . . '

Tall Boy interrupted me: 'Sometimes it's nice to be vulnerable.'

I looked at him and he smiled. Time will tell, I guess. We gave each other a peck on the cheek as we parted.

Friday 10th November

Tall Boy is away a lot, but he always has an interesting story about his travels. When we walk up to the high street together to get a sandwich for lunch or find something for the office I feel warm and protected in his company. I find his easy charm, kindly teasing voice and the stubble on his face so sexy, but strangely he never seems to be available for that drink I've been promising him for helping with my presentation.

He is off to France for the weekend. I wonder if he has a girlfriend there. I will have to wait for the right moment to ask.

Friday 17th November

Still no word from Cashmere, still so much activity on his dating profile. Maybe he was just logging on to check what I was up to? Somehow I doubt it; he must have been getting in touch with other girls and whisking them off on dates . . . showing them his naughty books . . buying them rings . . .

So, I did what any sensible woman would have done in my place, and set about creating an 'alternative profile' for him, which mentioned his arrogance, his coldness, his habit of leaving me hanging in mid air instead of telling me it was all over. Nothing really below his virtual belt – I may be psycho but I am fair. And I wanted to warn any other lonely hearts who might be wandering into his trap.

The dating site realised what had happened after a day or two, suspended my profile and sent me a snide note about their 'terms and conditions' so I let off a little steam by pointing out that Cashmere had broken some 'terms and conditions' too, by using others for sex and then ignoring them.

Sunday 3rd December

I have heart, mind and body set on Tall Boy but I have no idea if I have a chance.

Just sitting across the desk from him, laughing with him, riding on that tension is enough just now. He is intelligent, multilingual, always joking, and we practise our French, German and Spanish in the office. He is helpful and I can always come to him for assistance if I need a hand with something I am working on. He compliments me every time he sees me and seems interested in what I've been up to. Our occasional lunches together are fun and flirty, but I've not been able to dig deeper and go into his current domestic arrangements. I don't see the point in putting energy into anything else. When I like someone this much I'd want it to be the real thing, and not just some flash in the pan. My memory is too long – I don't want another disaster. Even BBP left me a little messed up emotionally, when we could have just had an uncomplicated, purely physical fling. I can't keep my emotions out of anything, it seems.

Either that or I've got some kind of selective frigidity.

However, I can't ignore how the office lights up with energy on the days he works here. His presence fills me with a warm glow that lasts all day and our banter makes me giggle until my cheeks hurt. When he shows me something he's working on and I get close to him to see his screen, my senses are taken on a spin by his scent. I love the presence of his body, so tall and strong – I inhale whenever he breathes out and the thought that my wrists would feel tiny in his hands makes my knees weak with desire. I'd love to touch his curly head like you'd touch a child's, but of course that wouldn't be too professional.

Monday 4th December

Home from work early after a Tesco's curry sabotaged my attempts to flirt foxily with Tall Boy over the printer – ten minutes (or maybe three hours) of vomiting in the only loo in the office didn't provoke any offer from him to see me safely home. He seemed concerned but didn't get involved, which disappointed me. What was I expecting? My fun, uncomplicated work colleague to suddenly morph into my knight in shining armour? Maybe a bit more initiative, that's for sure. 'Are you all right?' he asked when he came back from my boss's office to find my collapsed form on the sofa, looking very pale. 'Um, no,' I told him, embarrassed about my vulnerability. I can't expect him to just drop everything and walk me to the tube, knowing my boss's temper and the workload they have to get through. So I pretended I'd be OK and shuffled away, smelling of sick and feeling like my insides had turned to raw eggs. So much for Sienna, office seductress.

Wednesday 6th December

How to get over the fact that the man you like doesn't fancy you:

- Eat. This will make your endorphins rise, causing a temporary respite from a depressed mood, and it will also make you fat so that you become obsessed with your weight instead of silly men.
- Read sexy books, then wank. At least you know how to get yourself off.
- Put a random ad on a new internet site and flirt via MSN in the office while Tall Boy sits opposite you, minding his own business. Feel fabulous and reassured that he has no idea what he's missing.
- Don't invite him to join you for lunch for the second day in a row. If he wants to have lunch with you, let him do the asking. Similarly, stop asking him what he's up to at the weekend because he is always away. And no more 'friendly' invites for drinks – you only give him a chance to fob you off with some excuse.
- Go home early and watch DVDs. A deserved early night plus a leisurely wank will make you even more attractive the next morning, maybe causing him to change his mind.

At least I'm about to exchange on the flat, though. Fingers crossed.

Wednesday 13th December

I just realised that this will be my second single Christmas since Pinocchio, and now I'm sobbing violently. I made a pledge to myself after the break-up that I'd never take anyone home to meet my folks at Christmas again until they'd bought me a rock the size of a Ferrero Rocher, to make their intentions clear and save me from further embarrassment with the family.

There isn't even anyone to warm my bed. This is the same bed that saw me and BBP writhing in our own sweat, contorting into all sorts of positions and reaching orgasm after orgasm, his dreads in my face, the only words we swapped about the tightness of my pussy and the rightness of each caress.

I miss rolling over and hugging my Sweet Ex, the one before Pinocchio. He was too young when we got together and three and a bit years down the line, with him still living with his parents, I was running out of patience. In retrospect, I am almost regretting the split now because I lost that love and I am on my own.

I miss the warm, musty duvet in Pinocchio's bed, his head on my chest while he slept and I read my book, the cat resting on my feet.

I miss the annoying birds and the early morning light which crept across Cashmere's big white bed and looking across at his tangle of blond curls and catching his blue eyes' first glimpse of the day and me.

I miss being able to ring someone up just because they care how I am. I miss sharing the excitement of good news – my job! My flat! – and the frustrations of disappointments with someone.

Pathetic.

Have also decided to go off the Pill to see what my body does. I've been on it for so long to regulate my hormone levels (I have slightly raised testosterone thanks to PCOS) that I'm curious to see if I'll still ovulate, plus for years my 'week off' has always been marked by horrendous headaches. Surely it's better not to take it at all, especially now I am not in a relationship, than to take it and then have to swallow painkillers three days a month?

Later:

Determined to be less pathetic, I reminded myself about the ad I placed on a new site, saying 'Posh Boy wanted' (inspired by the memory of Cashmere's snooty accent and what it always did for me). I've had five responses so far . . .

Friday 15th December

All I want for Christmas:

- A game of 'Hard to Get' with full instruction leaflet.
- Stockings (Agent Provocateur).
- The film the Colonel shot of us dancing on the Côte d'Azure (fat chance).
- A set of blinkers (man-proof).
- A box of tissues (man-size).
- Something in a Tiffany's box.
- A version of The Sims where they actually get naked and have sex, not just stand opposite each other going 'woo hoo!'
- A discreet murder weapon to use on people listening to loud music and smoking on the bus.
- A job with half the hours and twice the pay.
- A shag.

Tuesday 19th December

After puking me, Tall Boy got to see blubbing me in the office. The bank's trying to make complications with my mortgage. I do not need this a few days before I go away for Christmas. So much stress I couldn't do anything but bawl my eyes out by lunchtime. I really hope I look cute when I cry, or Tall Boy will be scared off for good after seeing me snuffling and red-eyed, begging my current landlord for an extension on the tenancy.

Wednesday 20th December

When I get home from work tonight I'm going to be busy packing my suitcase and present-wrapping for Christmas, but now I can just make the time to write about my little seasonal pick-me-up.

I believe that coming off the Pill has made me hornier and more daring – without the artificial hormones, my testosterone is starting to kick back in. Out with the girls on Saturday I spotted an uncomfortable-looking guy in a jumper, who seemed out of place in the club. He was tall with a bit of a belly, but handsome despite his awkwardness. I kept seeing him around on trips to the dance floor or the bar, and eventually went up to him and introduced myself. We had a nice little chat and I teased him about the jumper, which he said was all the rage at trendy ski resorts this year. After a while a mate came to grab me and get me to dance, but I kept one eye on Jumper Boy.

My girl friends wanted to leave early but I wasn't tired yet, so when I saw Jumper Boy heading for the stairs to leave I caught up with him to either say goodbye or try and change his mind about calling it a night. He was easily swayed, looking pleased to be apprehended and we left right away. Climbing into a taxi I asked the driver to take us to a nearby cocktail bar, but it was closed, alas, so as I had no intention of being precipitously whisked back to his flat in Fulham or wherever, I suggested another club that I used to go to with Samantha.

For fun I led him through a little door into the tiny 'secret room' in the club, not much bigger than a large closet, with red velvet couches, a pole for dancing and saucy paintings on the walls of transvestites in fetish outfits having oral sex, or women in huge skirts being spanked.

Jumper Boy and I suckled massive champagne cocktails and had a very civilised conversation, despite the artwork, which obviously unsettled him a little. I don't think he realised that some clubs have rooms like this, and was surprised that I knew my way around them.

He kissed me abruptly and I was glad – imagine if I'd picked up a guy, closeted him in a secret sex room and then all he'd wanted was my sparkling conversation? We lay back on the couch, kissing more and more passionately until I got the giggles and asked if he even remembered my name. He paused and switched on his brain: 'Um . . . ' he said. 'I told you!' I laughed. 'So what's mine?' he asked me. And I got it right first time. He grinned and frowned. 'Your name begins with an S?' he probed. 'Yes . . . ' 'Oh, Sienna!' and I rewarded him with a kiss.

Making out in the secret room felt naughty and exciting. We could hear the music pumping out in the club and people's shouted conversations, laughter and the clink of glasses but we had absolute privacy. Or at least, almost – there was no lock for the door, and anyone could have walked in at any moment. Other clubbers probably thought the nondescript door was the entry to a broom cupboard or a staff-only part of the club.

Things got more heated. He slid a hand under the waistband of my jeans to caress my bum, and I could feel my pussy flooding with excitement. I wrapped my arms round him and scratched his skin a little, pulled his hair and sucked his lips. He pinned me onto the red velvet.

He tugged his hand round inside my jeans so he could wriggle his fingers down the front of my knickers, and when he felt how wet I was he quickly pulled his hand out and began to work at my flies, ready to pull my trousers down. I panicked a bit. Was he going to fuck me right there? Did he have a condom? He struggled to unzip his own trousers and I bent my head over his cock, surreptitiously sniffing it – it smelt clean and I closed my lips on it, intrigued by the shape of it – the shaft was long and the head huge.

After a few seconds he pushed me back and yanked at my jeans till they were round my ankles – the door was right behind him, ready to fling open and expose me to the gaze of some unwitting clubber. He tried to enter me but I pushed his head down and made him lick me. He didn't have much patience but it felt nice and made me want more.

'You got a condom?' I asked and he fumbled in his designer wallet for a little foil packet and handed it to me. I ripped it open but could see he was losing heart and hard-on, so quickly rolled it on him. He told me to turn and face the mirror on the back wall, then entered me from behind with relish. He bucked into me, his balls beating on my thighs, his cock rubbing at my G-spot . . . it felt great, and then it was over, way too soon, and he was buckling up his jeans and muttering about his white arse being on display to anyone. I could have spent half an hour there fucking, having forgotten to be self-conscious in favour of sheer fun.

'Why would anyone walk in? If a club has a private room I'm sure they know better than to barge in.' Then I started to tease him. 'There might be a camera though, or this could be a two-way mirror.'

He stuck the used condom in an empty cocktail glass and I tucked the wrapper behind one of the paintings and we walked nonchalantly out and into the main club, blasted by the music. 'I can't believe I had sex in a club!' he exclaimed excitely. 'I never thought I'd do that!' he kept on saying. I sat down in a booth and Jumper Boy trotted off to get more cocktails.

I took the opportunity to fleece the pocket of his Aquascutum coat – I'd just had sex with a man I knew nothing about, so I was entitled to feel nosey. Some sort of medical kit, a Razr phone and two Mars Bars. I twigged he must be a diabetic, although what he was doing drinking sugary cocktails and eating mince pies in the club, I have no idea. Hopefully he wouldn't fall into a coma now!

He brought back two completely awful drinks, so I suggested we leave – he still owed me an orgasm after all. We got a taxi back to his place, and he warned me about the state of it. It was a tip – he said he was doing it up and as there wasn't a bathroom he's using the kitchen sink instead. Shaving, washing up, brushing his teeth, filling the kettle, washing himself . . . Picking their way around the debris were two of the most adorable cats I'd ever seen.

I sat down on a sofa strewn with dirty pants and he played with the cats and made us bacon sandwiches, mentioning the need to keep his blood sugar levels up. It was three a. m. and we tore into the sandwiches – I hadn't eaten anything but mince pies and a few nachos since breakfast. There were masses of antique furniture he'd bought at auction or inherited, covered with junk and standing on filthy carpets. The cats were everywhere and it was quite a relief when he lit candles and switched off the lights.

We retired to bed where he tried to make an issue of the condom again because he 'doesn't like them'. Tough. I tried not to think about the implications – if he's that used to fucking bareback, doesn't that mean there's a steady girlfriend in the picture? I made him wrap up, and got my orgasm with a vengeance, via all my favourite positions, missionary, me on top and doggy style. I made as much noise as possible to wake up the neighbours.

Mission accomplished, I slept like a baby, snuggled in his arms, till five when the cats had a fight on my back. The next morning he was the perfect gent, making me Earl Grey as I sat on the sofa in one of his shirts, then coming to loll with me and throw things for the cats to chase. It started to feel like more than a one-night stand. We joked and kidded and he even told me some serious stuff about his family and life. He took me to a nearby café for breakfast and told me about his diabetes, injecting himself through his trousers in front of me – apparently he'd injected his own wallet more than a few times!

I had to leave and go to yet another Christmas party, so after he'd walked me to the tube where we kissed goodbye, I asked for his number. In return I got a Café Nero loyalty card which he scribbled his email address on.

'Oh. So is the seventh shag free?' I joked, and he laughed awkwardly. No number, eh? And no surname either.

Friday 22nd December

Up at the crack of dawn for my flight to my folks' this morning, although it was sweetened by getting a lift from my door to the airport. I haven't blogged about him, but I've been seeing a little of one of the guys who responded to my 'posh boy wanted' ad. We corresponded by email for ages and I was drawn in by his intelligence, wit and obvious desire for a meaningful relationship. The only problem was it took for ever to persuade him to send me a photo of himself, and when one did arrive it was grainy and he looked grumpy, which wasn't promising.

Even though I was late to our first date, he waited for me for nearly an hour, then when I'd made my profuse apologies he charmed me over dinner, even if I thought I didn't fancy him. I thought he was a little bit fat, to be honest, and a bit short for me – but I was just enjoying the conversation and the 'click'. He seemed mesmerised by me and I started to appreciate his green eyes and easy smile.

When I climbed into his car this morning there were three of the books we'd talked about over dinner waiting for me on the seat. I'd threatened to be a bit surly at that time in the morning but now I was smiling broadly about the books so he teased me, 'I'm disappointed you're not more grumpy.' And I forgot all about the fact that I'm not a morning person.

At least I've made a nice new friend, even if Jumper Boy is scared off by a minx with access to secret sex rooms and Tall Boy continues to remain indifferent to my charms. I shall call him Kensington Boy, KB for short.

Tuesday 2nd January 2007

New Year's Eve one-night-stand etiquette while staying with your mum:

+ Don't get drunk.
+ Don't forget to text her to let her know you're still alive at four a. m.
+ Try not to lose your house keys.
+ When she greets you at the door at ten a. m., near out of her mind with worry, try to act sympathetically.
+ Try to act sober.
+ Be vague about the number of people who were at the house you ended up at. Do not let slip that it was just two – you and the man whose surname you don't know.
+ Give the name of the man who dropped you off at the house as though he's been in your group of friends for ages, known him sooo long!

- Pretend he was sober when he drove you home.
- Say you lost your keys at the club.
- Attempt to cure early-onset cystitis from rampant sex-with-a-stranger by drinking baking soda in water, without your mother seeing you.
- Pretend to your sister's boyfriend that you thought the guy was older than twenty-four.
- Happy New Year!

Thursday 4th January

Kensington Boy picked me up from the airport in his sparkly car and we fell into conversation like old friends. I've got addicted to his intelligent, self-deprecating emails and brilliant writing, and I could get used to his reassuring presence, his conversation and his chauffeuring skills.

What else has been going on? What's going to happen in 2007? Well, the Pilot has blasted in from the past and asked to meet up 'for a coffee'. I shouldn't have put him on the email list about my flat purchase going through. Maybe he thinks I have money and can pay for his pilot's licence? Or maybe he misses the casual sex? I may meet up with him, or stand him up. Now there's a thought.

Rugby Boy has been in touch too. I haven't seen him since March. He now has that conservatory he'd been promising himself.

Nothing from Tall Boy.

Friday 12th January

I hadn't even kissed Kensington Boy and yet he lugged the entire contents of my old flat down two flights of stairs and into a van, rode across town with me, then lugged everything up two more flights of stairs into the new flat.

We were talking about relationships, and I moaned that whenever things go well (and I get spoiled) it all goes up in a puff of smoke. 'Would you rather be spoilt for a short time or not at all?' he asked me, cheekily, and I was stumped. How do you answer that? A little is better than none, I suppose, but if it could be heartache free, that would be even better. There needs to be some kind of back-up when your spoiling time is over, otherwise the world is a sad and lonely place.

So I asked him, 'Would you rather be dumped at the start, or after a short and debauched affair?' He picked the affair, with an option to follow-up friendship afterwards. 'It's an ego thing,' he explained, and I made a mental note.

Tuesday 16th January

I am being truly wooed. What would you say to someone who is falling for, and sleeping with, someone who looks a bit like a fat Hitler without the moustache? That was what I thought of KB when he pulled up outside my new flat in his 'ridiculously poncy' (his words) car, his bouncy hair brushed back and parted in the middle where it had dried after his morning shower.

Less than twelve hours after an exhausting trip to a large Scandinavian furniture store, I let his rotund form fuck my quivering body senseless, my head a mess of lust and emotions and my pussy already satisfied from his quick but effective dive between my thighs earlier (when I took the liberty of mussing up his hair to get rid of the Nazi do). I'd pounced on him after the last box of flatpack was safely in the door, desperate for him.

I'm not exactly *ashamed* of him, but I am a bit. Does that make sense? Does it make me a bad person? Much as I'm swooning for all his qualities, I can't help but wonder what people think when they see us walk down the street together. OK, I'm not the slimmest girl in zones 1–2 but I'm tall, blonde and coolly dressed and there he is with his well-cut suits and belly. Do they mentally chirp, 'She must be with him for his money'? He looks about ten years older than he is, thanks to the clothes and the gut, even though he's my toy boy by a couple of years.

What's my problem? Let's weigh up the pros and cons:

Pros:	Cons:
His ability to come to the rescue at any moment.	Oooh, about 2–4 stone.
He genuinely cares about me.	Umm.
	Yeah.
His touch is electric.	There must be something else?
He smells and tastes nice.	
He plies me with champagne in expensive restaurants.	His inability to wear t-shirts?
His wit and irony.	The fact I'm half a head taller than him in heels?
He wears cashmere but I don't think of Cashmere.	He can't dance or sing?
	That's it.
He really listens and remembers everything I say.	
He likes to surprise me with gifts.	
His writing.	
His ability to calm me down.	
His patience.	
He loves small kids.	
An old-fashioned gent.	
His maturity.	

Wednesday 17th January

Last night KB took me to his flat for the first time, more by coincidence than plan – we were both hungry and passing, and he said he'd tidied the place up. It's charmingly furnished, with books everywhere and fascinating knick-knacks and, on his wall, two framed photos of him with some girl.

I knew who she was immediately. The Ex.

And I got that horrible sinking feeling in the pit of my stomach as though I'd shot down in a lift from bliss to the basement. My hunger vanished and I just wanted to go home, preferably right away, before I cried. I just wanted to be conjured back to my own bedroom, alone, with my shopping, which was still in his car.

I've barely known him six weeks and I can't stake any claim to what he puts on his walls or to the contents of his heart, but this seemed like a cruel twist of fate. I've tried not to feel this vulnerable, not for twenty-two months, and I've failed quite often, but not for lack of trying. Here it was, staring me in the face.

I remember Pinocchio's ex, grinning at me from the fridge, the bookcase, the top of the chest of drawers, the hall table . . . of course, she 'had absolutely no significance' but if I hid the frames they'd reappear by my next visit, like magic.

'KB,' I tried to sound cheerful, 'who are the people in the pictures?'

'Oh, that's my brother, and that's my dad and mum, and that's my nan, and, oh, that's me and my ex.'

His kisses made me prickle the wrong way. I ate the meal he'd cooked and drank the wine, making small talk and trying to regain my appetite while her irritating mug stared down at the back of my neck from the wall.

'I have this silly rule,' I finally said, as he wrapped me in his arms and kissed me again, 'but may I have another piece of bread first?' He looked puzzled as he went to slice the bread and watched me eat it in silence. He hazarded a guess and got it wrong and started to look crestfallen, as if he thought I'd turned cold on him.

'I don't sleep with men in flats where there are still pictures of their exes on the wall.'

He was shocked when he realised what the photos were signalling, and I felt my eyes were welling up and tried to crack a joke about something else. He told me they 'didn't mean anything' and he just hadn't gotten round to taking them down yet – everything I'd heard from Pinocchio. Word for word. But then he said, 'You know, if I saw her now she'd cross the street to avoid me,' whereas Pinocchio had said, 'She's like a sister.'

I tried to tell him not to worry so much about me, and excused myself to the loo, where I did some deep breathing and calmed myself down.

When I went back into the living room he showed me two cupped palms full of ripped-up photos which he stuffed in the bin in a grand gesture, dusting his hands as he was done.

I let him drive me home and succumbed to his amazing hands and tongue again. As my walls are still bare of photos I managed to clear my head long enough to come three times and chuck him out just before two a. m.

Neurotic, moi?

Tuesday 23rd January

Images of my lover that I can't shake today:

- His hands on my thighs and my arse in the club, feeling for my suspender belt and stocking tops.

- His face cracking into a smile as I caress his cheeks with velvet gloves.
- His hand on the small of my back, penetrating me with warmth and possessing me.
- Caressing my thighs and stocking tops in the car, pushing my skirt up, regardless of the cyclists whizzing past the windows and the street lights beaming down.
- Feeling his way into my knickers while he steers with one hand.
- His gruff voice telling me I have no choice but to screw him.
- His finger in my pussy, tongue on my clit, stubble around my labia.
- His breath, his smell (I could even smell his pre cum when he was still in his suit).
- Him bending me over, me in nothing but seamed stockings and suspenders, him in dress shirt, black Armani trousers and braces.
- Him telling me he'll force me if I resist, and insisting he really will.
- Grasping my wrists and grabbing my hips.
- One of my hands on the floor, the other on my clit.
- Putting the condom on with my mouth, him telling me he'd make me suck his cock all day.
- His hands on my bare bottom, squeezing, pushing his cock inside.
- Him pushing into me, us rolling on the floor to avoid the squeaky bed.
- Pounding me, his breath hot in my ear.
- Slight slap on my bare bottom.
- Wiping the sweat off my shoulders.

- Coming, coming inside me.
- Collapsing and holding me.
- Telling me he thinks the world of me.
- The world.

Still in his suit.

Wednesday 24th January

I had my housewarming party last night and invited both Tall Boy and KB, because, well, why not? I do still fancy Tall Boy but I'm smitten with my posh lover. Tall Boy got a bit drunk on the cocktails KB made with my contraband holiday rum (so much for the man who says he never drinks them) and they engaged in some sort of subtle cockfight. Tall would jokingly punch the wall, macho fashion, and KB would solicitously refill my glass, hovering nearby, holding my hand. They engaged in a bit of competitive banter too, then Tall Boy tried to persuade my new lodger to come clubbing 'till the cows come home' – but she stayed in regardless.

To be honest, I didn't care if Tall Boy snogged her, or if he saw me holding hands with KB, or the way KB was acting the host, fetching drinks and taking coats – Tall Boy's been so flaky. And KB knows how to act like a man and a gent to boot. Although I did feel like telling him to just relax and let people get their own drinks.

Everyone took their shoes off which had the unexpected bonus that when people spilled their drinks their socks soaked it up.

Nicola left early and as she was pulling her shoes on in my bedroom, she just had to make a stab at KB's appearance. 'Sienna, seriously – *him*?' she asked me in a whisper. She had seen us holding hands and didn't get it. 'Yes, I like him,' I told her, annoyed at the criticism. 'He is sweet, intelligent, really helpful, he can cook, I love talking to him . . . ' 'Sure, but in the *bedroom*?' she made it sound like I was sleeping with King Kong. 'All great,' I snapped, peeved at her shallowness. Did she think he had hypnotised me into going out with him? Surely she wouldn't have been so negative if he'd been some six-foot Adonis without a brain. Why can't she just be happy for me?

Following Nicola's departure I led everyone off down the street and on to a club, carrying plastic cups of booze, leaving Tall Boy to sweet-talk my flatmate, and made them all play 'I have never'.

I confessed everything.

'I have never had sex this week,' someone said. I drank.

'I have never had sex on a yacht.' I drank again.

'I have never had sex in a club.' 'What kind of club?' I asked the laughing crowd, then drank again. KB drank on 'I have never had sex with a man', but when I pressed him he said he'd just been thirsty. Ha!

'I have never had sex for seven days in a row' – that threw us all into a few seconds of silence while we wracked our memories. 'Wouldn't you get cystitis on day five?' I asked, sacrilegiously, and got everyone laughing again.

Cheers! Here's to new flats and new loves!

Later:

The Pilot just phoned to try and 'nail down' that coffee. I didn't have his number stored in my phone so was surprised to hear his voice, then had to explain to him that I'd deleted it. We had a pleasant chat and might see each other when he's finished his latest training week.

Thursday 25th January

This morning I woke up happily between KB's designer sheets, and made my way to his en-suite wearing his size XL Ralph Lauren pyjamas. He'd gotten up earlier and I'd thought he was in the lounge, but he was standing in the bathroom with the lights off – maybe he had a wee in the dark so the lights wouldn't wake me? Who knows, but I was so startled that I screamed, then slipped on the wet floor, and he reacted in an instant, grabbing me by the lapels and pulling me into a hug to reassure me. I pressed my nose into his bathrobe, which smelt of him and his shaving foam.

I felt calmed and happy, and then surprised at myself because we'd gone to bed late and after a slightly rocky evening, following a confession by me. Which is worse? Avoiding younger men because they don't want to settle down and you do, or telling the younger man you're sleeping with that you shouldn't be sleeping with people who aren't serious because you have decided that you've had enough of the casual dating scene and want to settle down and have babies?

The realisation that my heart gets involved every time my pussy is having some action surprised me, and confessing it to someone I'd only been seeing a few weeks was almost a shock, but his reaction reassured me. He stayed calm and listened, holding me and stroking my back without freaking out at the crying woman in his bed.

My sudden mood change had been caused by a dip in endorphins because I'd missed my orgasm. Every few seconds that we fucked, KB would check that the condom was still in place, a manoeuvre that killed the mood and made me frustrated. Stop-starting every few seconds when I'm this close, *this close* to an orgasm . . . My patience wore thinner than any Durex.

To think that such a wonderful, sweet and decent, intelligent individual has a total obsession with the grip of his condom whilst the world's biggest bastards procreate like flies thanks to their emotional latex allergies!

I rolled over when he'd come and lay there feeling awful. He was concerned and then apologetic and heard me out. I cheered up and it was all right. He says he does want kids, but he's too conscientious (or sober) to attempt even a little bit of risky sex, and now that caution has robbed me of an orgasm.

8

Be My Baby

WINTER/SPRING 2007

Tuesday 30th January

I am so happy.

Funny that. You know, all KB's amazing qualities are rolled up in a body you'd never see gracing the cover of a superficial magazine, but I am blissfully, bubblingly falling in love with him.

He came round on Saturday to help me look after the little boy I sometimes baby-sit and we had loads of fun at the playground and at the swimming pool in 'baby soup' with all the other kids, even though KB says he's neither sporty nor fond of water. He was great with the little one and seemed to enjoy himself genuinely.

I got a bit sentimental when a thought hit me all of a sudden: 'I've always wanted kids before I'm thirty,' I said sadly to KB, 'and now I just realised that won't happen.' 'You'll make a great mummy,' he told me, watching me affectionately with my friend's son.

We dried off and went back to mine for some food, then watched the telly until the child's mother came to pick him up. Then us grown-ups went to bed, even though it was only tea time.

He eased my jeans and knickers off and went down on my chlorinated pussy for ages, then I returned the favour, before we had a good, lusty fuck, me loving the sound of him slapping against me, and the fact that he's not as gentle as he used to be. He deposited a large amount of sticky cum on my arm and belly and we cuddled for a while before getting ready for a friend's party that evening.

He drove and I read the map and swigged from a little bottle of cheap fizzy wine, listening to Unknown FM and cracking jokes all the way. The party was subdued but fun – one couple had even brought their dog along, and there was a French boy at the 'bar' making a mean Mojito – but after I'd fallen down the stairs in my fuck-me boots and KB had nearly gotten stoned from passive smoking, we decided to call it a night.

Sunday morning was lovely: a long, lazy wake-up fuck and more talking before breakfast and a shopping trip, and he turned out to be as much of a bargain hunter as I am. That evening, as promised, he'd made me chocolate mousse (with real chocolate!) which we consumed on the sofa, clutching a champagne flute each. He massaged my feet and we talked and made love till two a.m. I slipped his brand-new trousers and a pink tie on over my bra and knickers, and discovered that my hip size is the same as his waist when he whipped the trousers off in one.

On Monday morning I opened one eye to see him looking at me lying on my back, and said,

'I'm still asleep, and you have just climbed in the window. Now you are trying to seduce me without waking me.' Then shut my eye again. I felt the mattress shift as he positioned himself over me and began to trail his fingers along my skin and over my arse, so gently that it felt like a trail of goose bumps were following his touch, then he pushed his fingers between my legs, and slowly dipped one into my pussy before twirling it round my clit and kissing my nipples as he touched himself.

He rubbed his erect cock against my thighs, and then, making me flood, against my cunt, kneeling between my legs as I went on 'sleeping'.

'The intruder wants to fuck you,' he said, 'don't you think you might wake up?'

'I might, or I may just think it's all an amazing dream.'

What a nice start to the week. And I wasn't even late to work.

Tuesday 6th February

The ex reared her ugly head, sending me into a downward spiral of depression. I cried down the phone to KB, to my mum and off the phone to nobody in particular. I hung about in the office for an extra hour alone because I didn't want to cycle home with my sight blurred by tears. Then I got crisps, dips, asparagus and a bottle of special-offer plonk from Tesco and settled in front of the telly to watch *Ugly Betty*. I didn't bother to cook the asparagus, just dipped it and crunched through it.

KB arrived to find the bottle mostly empty and me mostly full. I don't think anything I said made much sense. All I knew was that the next morning he was going to be meeting his ex to give her back a chair and other odds and ends. Normal stuff really, but it all got blown out of proportion by my Pinocchio'd brain, the bit I try to keep locked up most of the time.

KB coaxed me and massaged my feet until I nearly tore his clothes off him and we made sweet, sweaty love accompanied by creaky bed slats and animal noises (I was too drunk to be considerate for the neighbours and too turned on to care). *Ugly Betty* ended and I passed out before remembering to puke up the wine. Woke at two a. m. still in my knickers (KB didn't bother to remove them or his own boxers in the heat of the moment . . .)

Saturday he saw the ex then came back to me for more shopping and fucking, and we tried to go to a bar in his neighbourhood, but his post-shag hair was so bad that the staff seemed to think we were invisible, so we went to a more questionable establishment down the road.

You had to ring a bell and wait for admission, and then descend a flight of stairs to a basement where there was mid-nineties music, a rather drunk bloke and two tarts, one in a low-cut top and the other a gold lamé mini-dress. They didn't have half the ingredients for the drinks on the menu, and when we finally picked the right cocktails the barman filled them up with watery ice. Every man who came in gave me a rather strange, inquisitive look – or three. What was this place?

KB and I, whispering to each other in a corner, clearly weren't the correct clientele, so after a drink and a half we went home to fuck and fall asleep in each other's arms.

Sunday was an emotional rollercoaster. KB was up before me and went to the lounge to read cookbooks while I slept on, sprawled diagonally across his Ralph Lauren sheets. After my second consecutive dream about Nazis, work, or other unpleasant subjects I got up to join him, snuggled on the sofa in his too-big pyjamas. I felt a bit sick, but my stomach improved after he brought me Buck's Fizz with freshly squeezed orange juice, ground coffee beans for cappuccino and whipped up a full English breakfast. All I had to do was smile (no problem, I was so happy), look pretty and read a book about a botched sex-change operation. Easy really.

Radio 1 began playing my favourite song from a previous summer holiday and I stripped off his pyjama top and gave him a little performance of the dance routine me and my gay friends had come up with that year. I bounced about in the sunlight with my boobs out for half the neighbourhood to see. The boy lives in a fish bowl but I don't care.

He was a very appreciative audience and I was rewarded with an invitation, 'Would you like to join me in the bedroom?' in my favourite husky voice, his hands between my thighs.

On the bed I straddled him and he eagerly pushed himself into me. I rocked and rode him till he exploded inside me, I collapsed on top of him with my fingers pressed against my clit, our first simultaneous orgasm.

Later, back at my flat, I began to wonder why I had woken up feeling ill, which was weird because I hadn't had much to drink the night before, and I still didn't have my period. KB helped me hang my curtain rail, but I suddenly got so dizzy standing on the chair with the drill that I had to sit down.

'Let me do it,' he offered, climbing onto the chair, and I watched with concern because I was sure it would collapse under his weight.

As the day went on, that weird dizzy feeling didn't subside and just before we got to the cinema that evening, I wondered aloud to him why I hadn't felt much like drinking the night before. I couldn't concentrate on anything, because I was suddenly convinced I was pregnant. We hadn't had any accidents with the condoms, but sometimes you don't need to break one to have a slip, especially when he keeps going soft.

KB noticed that I seemed quiet and asked me what was wrong: 'I just worry about what any boy would worry about when his girlfriend is feeling off-colour,' he said, so I admitted that that's what I'd been thinking too, even though

I felt embarrassed to have had the same thought. 'My period is usually fairly regular,' I said, but thinking that maybe my cycle had still not re-established itself properly since I came off the Pill. He just took my hand and said he'd stick by me. He was so calm and collected, even when I piped up in a small voice that we'd only known each other less than three months, and then he came right out and told me he was bringing in enough money to look after a family, and I shouldn't worry.

He suggested getting a pregnancy test and we drove across town to an all-night pharmacy so we could put my mind at rest. When we got back to my flat and the test turned out to be negative, I was shocked at how disappointed I felt. KB in comparison seemed very relieved for someone who'd been so unperturbed at the thought of fatherhood.

And I got my period this morning.

Here's a list of reasons why I never got pregnant by an ex:

◆ 'You are fit to have children', but as I was all of nineteen I freaked out and got the morning-after-pill. Twice. (Violent first boyfriend, 1997)

◆ 'Let me come on your back/tummy/tits/face . . . ' (anyone, any year)

◆ 'You will never find a twenty-three-year-old guy who will marry you and want to have kids.' (Sweet Ex, 2004)

◆ 'Not until I'm a millionaire! Public school costs £12,000 a term!' (Pinocchio, 2005)

◆ 'I am not ready yet.' (Dodgy thirty-eight-year-old boyfriend, 1999)

◆ 'If you are pregnant we are fucked.' (I'd told him I'd forgotten my Pill but he still didn't use a condom.

This from a man who'd already paid for two ex girlfriends' abortions: Pinocchio, 2005)

♦ 'I can't believe she got a degree in chemistry and then
got pregnant. She is wasting her education.' (Said
Porsche Boy of a married friend with a very sweet
baby and number two on the way)

♦ 'Babies are noisy, smelly and expensive.' (Said
Pinocchio, who thought nothing of spending £100 on
champagne and sundries, snored like a chainsaw and
only brushed his teeth when prompted)

♦ 'I am about to spend three years and £50,000 on
becoming a commercial pilot.' (The Pilot, 2005)

♦ 'I have herpes.' (The Sailor, 2005)

Ah well, no loss there, then . . .

Thursday 15th February

I had to work in the evening on Valentine's Day (don't ask – my
boss has bad timing for big projects) and I'd been paranoid
about asking KB what we'd do, not wanting to sound too much
like a clingy girlfriend, but even though he said the day was
overrated and tacky, he treated me to a champagne lunch.

When I was done at work at midnight he picked me up in his
car with a bottle of fizz and drove me home to 'molest me on the
sofa'. He told me he'd been having some little fantasies about me
all weekend and when I bent over the arm rest and offered him
my bum, he thrust in and said, 'That was one of them.'

He'd been worried that we didn't have any condoms, because
he thought that women ovulate right after their periods, but I
put him straight. I know my body pretty well and have always felt
my ovulation, to the point that I know which ovary is releasing

the egg. As well as counting the fourteen to fifteen days from the beginning of my period, I closely monitor the hormonal changes my body goes through by keeping an eye on my secretions. One of my parents' books explained this pretty well, and I am aware that drier, white mucus that sticks to my fingers and won't pull apart indicates a time that is safe from conception, whereas the days I can pull clear slime wide between my fingers mean I am fertile. KB probably has a point about wanting to be safe though, and I need to respect this. I expected him to pull out just before coming but then I could feel him building up then spewing his load deep into me. A divine feeling, but oh so wrong.

Last year on Valentine's Day I was seeing Cashmere, and that was the day he told me he didn't mind if I had other lovers. The year before that was Pinocchio, when I was blocking out a growing sense of unease. He cooked convenience food for me at home on the thirteenth, then cooked for his ex on the fourteenth, when I thought he was working. He crowned our celebration by calling me by her name. I got over it by eating the M&S roast and giving him a champagne blow job. Who said romance is dead?

Friday 16th February

I meant to write, but I forgot and I'm tired. There are now three sets of keys on my key ring:

My own.
The office's.
KB's.

A work contact invited me and a plus one to an exclusive midnight concert at Ronnie Scott's last night. I went home to rest (but ended up nattering to a friend on the phone), changed into a silk evening dress and hold-up stockings, then met KB in Soho. We were shown to our seats and he ordered me a glass of pink Moët. He couldn't take his eyes off me, or his hand off my knee.

As he slid his hand higher, tracing the bumps of my stocking tops through the silk and higher still, I tried to stop him.

'Everyone will see what you're doing by the position of your arm,' I warned him.

'But you love it, really.'

True. I was wet already.

When we got back to his he steered me straight from the taxi to his bedroom. My dress flew off over my head and I stood there in lacy knickers, a strapless bra, stockings and heels. He was eating me up with his eyes, his hands caressing my buttocks as he manoeuvred me onto the bed. I kicked my shoes off as he tugged my knickers away and pushed my legs apart, then stood back to strip his own clothes off hastily, fumbling the buttons. I unhooked my bra and reached for my faux-fur wrap to pull it round me. 'All furs and no knickers,' he remarked, and buried his head between my thighs.

I lolled back, caught between loving the way he gave me head, and frustration that it kept him away from me – he seemed miles away; all I could see was his face and his hair. Mind you, it's a nicer view than a set of dangling balls – Porsche Boy's favourite sixty-nine position (remember him?)

KB likes me to grab his head and push against his face, and I came pressing his face into my bare pussy, squirming with ecstasy. I love the feeling of his stubble on the tender flesh, so primeval, the horniest thing. He complimented me on my taste – why do men always say that? What do other girls taste like?

Am I a strawberry in a sack of potatoes, a juicy, sweet, pleasant surprise? – and fucked me to a second orgasm, his back sweating with the effort. Then he wrapped me up in his pyjamas and stroked me to sleep.

This morning he laid on the full works for breakfast and I was two hours late to work. Ah well. Boss wasn't in . . .

Saturday 17th February

The other night we made love while watching *Secretary*. He has taken to spanking me lightly if I ask him, and sometimes if I don't.

I want him to totally lose himself when he fucks me, to let me feel his weight, for him not to hold back, to use me, to be unrestrained and to restrain me. We play at words: 'What if I didn't let you?'

'What if I tried to anyway?'

'What if I tried to push you off?'

'What if you couldn't?'

He always reassures me he wouldn't do anything I didn't want him to, which spoils the fantasy somewhat, but sometimes he takes being masterful further than I've ever known it, and I like it.

'I want you to suck my cock,' he instructs.

'When?' I ask, pushing him.

'Now,' he answers curtly. I ask him to say please, and he does. Ha!

Sometimes he grabs my hair when I go down on him. He rubs his cock into my pussy, across my clit, teasing me and getting us both wet. He won't let me tell him when to enter me. He likes the suspense. Sometimes I touch him lightly, teasing him. He gets harder than if I yank or squeeze. He does lose his erection with condoms though . . .

Yes, we're occasionally now doing the dirty without condoms when it's 'safe'. It's much less frustrating than him going soft all the time and pulling the condom up. We've both been tested. We're OK. I know it's stupid, or is it? All nice things are stupid. Eating chocolate. Riding on a scooter without a helmet. Wearing a skirt when you're riding a horse. Swimming at night.

Sunday 18th February

I wish that intimacy didn't make me want to run a mile; I wish I could put all my eggs, emotional and physical, in one basket and feel at ease.

Am I ready to spend all that time with one person? Can the bliss overcome the fear? Why don't I look up the Sailor, or have that coffee with the Pilot, or answer one of Rugby Boy's texts with something more flirtatious? I'm courting disaster.

Some boy I gave my number to a while back has been texting, but I haven't answered. Yet. I wasn't really interested in him but now I think I should do something.

What's Cashmere up to? Has he moved on to a different girl? Most probably. Or a boy. My inner stalker suggests watching outside his house, or ringing the door bell. I had a dream where I went to a party at his house while he was away, and his flatmates and friends all welcomed me in, and I snooped around the place and mingled with the crowd. I felt oddly abandoned when I woke up.

Last time I was at KB's he popped out and left me to my own devices, and I jokingly threatened to look the place over. I did. I found a notebook but had trouble deciphering the handwriting in it. I thought one entry was titled 'wank phantasies' but then I looked again and it said, 'work meetings'.

My stomach dropped as I poked around and pried, but not the way it did when I uncovered Pinocchio's dirty secrets. I know I'm a bad, bad girl, but I've been burned before and now I'm looking for the smoke and the fire escape.

Monday 19th February

KB and I fucked the day away yesterday. Literally. We did it on my bed in the morning, and then, because I could hear my flatmate sneezing and coughing next door, on a duvet on the floor to spare her the bed creaking. I lost count of the number of orgasms I had. I fell asleep in his arms until lunch time, when he cooked me breakfast.

I felt so close to him, constantly touching, kissing, talking, his eyes filled with so much love and emotion that I had to make a silly comment and laugh it off before I said something deeper. I felt like melting. I ran a bath after breakfast, and welcomed him covered in a fur of bubbles, then set about massaging him and tickling him with pumice and he fucked me so gently that not a drop spilled over.

Then I turned on the shower and presented him my bare behind and we screwed standing under the jet, kneeling, standing, slipping a little on the sides of the bath. Then we threw a towel over the rug and fucked there, me looking up at the underside of the sink, sandwiched between the hard floor and his soft heaviness, our skin still wet and the shower running cold. I was slippery with so many orgasms and swollen from so many fucks already, and when he pushed himself roughly into me without even hesitating for a condom, he fucked me hard with the gentlest look on his face. I didn't want him to stop. I came again, and he withdrew and orgasmed.

The more I get to know him the more I like him, and the

more I find we have in common – our experiences, our attitudes, our expectations. I talked my friend's ear off telling her about KB, and probably bored her stupid.

Only I *must not* let him knock me up. I agree, I'm acting irrationally, we're not in the 'proper framework' to be doing this and I'm an irresponsible, daft woman for letting my hormones carry me away. I want to go back on the Pill. I don't want to go back on the Pill. But I'm getting frustrated with this fiddly business with condoms and erections that wilt when you produce them, and the fact that he only came twice in the two days of rampant shagging. I want him to come seven times too.

Tuesday 20th February

'Having a child together is a lifetime commitment, it's just not the right time yet,' he told me on the phone. 'If I said "let's get married tomorrow" you'd run a mile.'

'Give me some credit here,' I chuckled. The thought appealed to me, but obviously not to him. I'd just suggested we stop sleeping together, seeing as it confuses me so much.

'Is this the "let's just be friends" moment?' he asked.

'Nooooo!'

'Thing is,' he went on, 'as much as I don't want to screw you every time I see you, we end up doing it anyway.'

'Yes, you can't help it.'

Me neither.

Monday 26th February

'I love you just the way you are,' he said over dinner at his club when I made a remark about my figure and dessert.

'You what?' I kept my eyes on my plate.

'I love you just the way you are,' he repeated, louder, while I stared at my smoked salmon slipping slowly off my fork.

'I see,' I replied, with the biggest grin ever.

Later, when he was in me up to the hilt he whispered in my ear:

'What's your dirtiest fantasy?'

'I couldn't possibly tell you.'

'Go on . . . '

'What if . . . ' I kept my true dirtiest fantasy to myself and found another, 'What if you came into your club's library and found me there, pinned down by three men who offered me to you.'

'I would send them out.' Too polite.

'What if I struggled, and you needed them to hold me down?'

'I still wouldn't want them there,' he insisted.

'What if there was another guy here and I was blowing one of you while the other one fucked me – which one would you want to be?'

'The one who fucks you.'

'You could watch me sucking the other guy's cock . . . '

'Yes,' he grunted, thrusting harder.

Switching positions I rolled above him and lowered myself back onto his cock and the condom. 'What if some girl came and sat on your face, would you like that? I could kiss her for you.'

'Would you be jealous?'

I smiled and came. Well yeah, I thought to myself. Which is why this is fantasy, not reality.

Tuesday 27th February

Last week KB took me to a rather stiff and pretentious reception in honour of his old school, then on to his gentleman's club for dinner – always a grand affair, though I felt more comfortable there than I had before. He made me laugh by signing me in with the fake name I'd used in my first emails to him, and the waiter recognised me and was very sweet.

We ordered some lovely food and a half bottle of champagne so he could spoil me – it wasn't even the weekend. How decadent! Then we skipped pudding and retired to the library with some drinks.

I sat in the same huge leather armchair I sat in on an early date, before we'd even kissed and when there was so much sexual tension in the air. That time he only just stopped being shy enough to stroke my arm lightly. This time he was bolder.

Coming round behind me he forcefully kissed my neck and face, then slipped his hand into my top and caressed my nipple with his rough finger tips. It sprang to attention immediately and I felt myself gushing at the thought of one of the waiters coming in and surprising us. I didn't want him to stop. My eyes were scouring the room for alcoves, or long table cloths or secret doors so we could consummate this little flirtation. I could tell he was excited too, though not hard. He pushed my skirt up with his right hand, still pinching my nipple with his left, and put it firmly between my legs. Mildly scandalised and majorly turned on, I cried out in protest, despite not wanting him to stop.

He pulled his hands away. 'They'll ban me if they discover my guest in a state of undress in the library,' he teased. 'You even have to be married to share a bedroom here.'

I pulled my knickers down to give him a quick flash of my pussy, and then straightened my skirt, crossed my legs and sipped my drink demurely. Maybe we won't act out the fantasy this time.

Be My Baby

This morning I had a nightmare. I dreamt KB had gotten back together with his ex and I found them together, cuddled up with no space for me. He acted all aloof and told me he 'had to give it another go' with her. I cried, then planned my impotent revenge – impotent because I can't change someone else's heart. She was, of course, posher than me, posher than him even. I woke up early and couldn't go back to sleep.

Is this a warning dream, like the ones I had about Pinocchio's ex? I didn't go to sleep unhappy. Well, not really. I'd had a confusing weekend which was a mixture of blissful sex and coupledom with KB, and then being left alone when he'd gone home because of his cold, and leaving countless messages on friends' answerphones to see if they wanted to hang out with me and getting no response. What was he up to the rest of the weekend? Am I losing friends because I'm so wrapped up in him? I wish I wasn't such an attention junkie and could spend my time with nice, non-sexual friends instead of seeking reassurance by chasing cock.

He broke up with his ex in November. We started emailing each other in December.

I prefer having him at my place – a clean slate, no memories. I think of her body in his bed, his shower, on his sofa, her eating from the same plate that my lovingly cooked breakfasts are served on. Her legs around his head, her clothes in a drawer somewhere, her hand on the key that now hangs on my key ring.

Mindfuck. Sometimes I wish there was an off switch for my brain. It'd be easier to be stupid and have no imagination. This abandonment crap keeps playing itself out again and again in my head and my life. I need a way out.

Thursday 1st March

Today I deliberately dressed up for the office, for Tall Boy. Is this a bad thing? I wanted to look nice for him, despite the despicable weather and despite the fact that he's seen me with KB and told me he thinks he's a decent chap, and despite the way he's given me *no* encouragement to fancy him at all, if you don't count the cheeky looks he shoots me from his emerald eyes and the way he teasingly winds me up.

The thing is, he thinks we have nothing in common.

He likes Rock, I like House. He likes beer, I like champagne cocktails. He likes going to scruffy places with his mates and getting hammered, I like glam venues and civilised weekends that he finds pretentious. But why should any of that matter?

He has continually refused any suggestions that we go out again, although he did once text me at four in the morning when he was 'in my area' (and I was asleep next to KB) and called me one night about a party, which he then missed. When I was sick in the office he didn't even walk me to a taxi.

Does this make me superficial? He doesn't behave in a particularly nice way to me, and yet I'm in thrall to his looks and charm. But then again, KB has thrown all my expectations about looks and weight out of the window because even though he's short, fat and hairy, he makes my spine (and other places) tingle with lust and my head spin with his wit and intellect. He really is something special. I enjoy my lunches with Tall Boy, but I'm not sure what his other issues are. He recently mentioned cleaning out his house and how much of his ex's stuff he still found lying around. By the sounds of it, they settled down too soon and it didn't end well. I'll have to try and get around to asking him about it some day, as there seems to be more behind it. This could be an explanation for his constant attempts to live his bachelor life to the full, and his reluctance to acquire a girlfriend – maybe he's been hurt just as I have?

Friday 2nd March

In any relationship, if things are going to go forward and you're going to get more involved, there are little niggles that you have to consider – and eliminate. Ideally the cons are outweighed by the pros. Here are mine:

Ideally – he would have a raging hard-on as soon as things got 'interesting'. This boner would not subside until he has received a blow job, gone down on me and given me a thorough rogering (i.e. him going down on me, then sliding himself up my body and into me without interruption, just before I come, then fucking me vigorously until we have a simultaneous orgasm).

In reality – he doesn't always stay hard. When he does, he takes ages to come. This problem is directly related to condoms, which often seem to stop him coming at all, or cause him to go soft. Sometimes it takes for ever for me to get him hard, and I'm yanking and wanking away for ages.

Fortunately, he doesn't care if he doesn't come, although I do and it leaves me feeling frustrated and unsexy. He always makes sure I do get my orgasm, be it with a vibrator, two fingers, or his tongue. He won't continue fucking me if I've come and want to stop. He is extremely affectionate and says, 'It will sort itself out. Sorry. That's just me.'

I wonder if it's something to do with his ex.

Actually, now I'm feeling rather silly and am glad I wrote this down. I should have no cause for concern and just be happy when I'm with him. I like him a lot, I lust after him like crazy and he spoils me like a princess. So niggling voices, shut up!

Saturday 3rd March

I confessed my broodiness to Jess in an email, and she typed back, 'What's the rush? Don't women have babies in their sixties nowadays?'

Well, maybe some of them do, but I don't want to be one of them. That, and, well, I have a few medical issues that mean it's going to be hard for me to conceive, and harder still when I pass the age of thirty-four when all the scientists say your fertility begins to plummet. So that only leaves me a few years to get started, especially if I want to have more than one child.

And I've known I want them for years. I've always been around children, I've spent twenty-two years looking after them for other people. It's been more intense in the last three years – the longing in the pit of my stomach is about as far away from my intellect as it's possible to be. When I was all loved up with Sweet Ex I seriously considered it, although I'm glad I didn't now, otherwise I'd have had a child with a child, and that baby would have two broke parents.

So there *is* a rush, actually, especially when I wasted three and a half years on Sweet Ex, nine months on Pinocchio and now two more years trying to sort the wheat from the chaff with these lovers. Not an easy task at the best of times, especially when your judgement is clouded by the need for affection and bad memories of the past, and your over-active imagination lets you view your suitors through the rosiest of rose-tinted glass. No wonder I can't silence the niggling voices.

Wednesday 7th March

KB has been away with his dad to look at property abroad, but I haven't heard from him at all. Not even a text. Maybe his phone doesn't work abroad, but his dad must have one that does – he's got a wife and two toddlers at home. Did KB forget to take my number? That doesn't make any sense. Five days. Five whole days, after a blizzard of phoning and texting and cosiness and passion.

It brings up a rather nasty taste in my mouth, which is horrible enough because I'm recovering from one of the most evil stomach bugs known to woman ('Oh, maybe it's morning sickness!' I thought excitedly, even though I'd been changing tampons for the past three days).

Now I'm back at work, sick as a dog and driving myself crazy with obsessive thoughts, making a date with that random Asian bloke who kept on texting, and considering chasing up Jumper Boy from the club's 'secret room'. Anything to stop replaying those last few weeks with Pinocchio – finding the photos of him and the ex on the holiday they took in Spain, while I was at home, diligently feeding his stupid cat. Also, the memory of sending that picture of my pussy to Cashmere in New York and getting no reply – New York being the city where his ex lived. Never seeing Cashmere again and dreaming of him all the time . . .

I know that if I'm jealous and insecure I could drive KB away; my few months with him are nothing compared to eighteen months with his ex. But still, five days?

Friday 9th March

I went on a date last night. With that random bloke.

When I got home after work KB had already called twice and left messages with my flatmate. I checked my mobile, and yup, he'd called that too. Twice. No message though. I ignored it and got ready to go out, fuming but relieved he wasn't dead after all. To be honest, I wasn't exactly full of enthusiasm for the date with Random Bloke, but I had to do something to keep me from exploding.

I waited for him for ages at Euston, before phoning Random and demanding the name of the restaurant, like a diva: 'The station is cold and it smells. I can't wait here much longer.' Turns out he was in the station waiting for me, at another exit.

He was falling over himself to apologise to me about the wait, and tremendously sweet. We found the restaurant and had some nice food, the conversation flowing easily. We talked about our cultural backgrounds, families, careers, flats, the things we like to do, etc etc etc. All I could think about was KB. I asked Random if he'd had any interesting dates lately. He said no, and asked me the same.

'Remember what I said before, that I'm sort of seeing someone?' I launched into an explanation of how that didn't stop me meeting other men for dinner, since I wasn't in a committed relationship. Random seemed to agree, although I couldn't help feeling rubbish about it.

This boy didn't deserve to have his time wasted by a girl who had given her heart away to another man. And KB might not deserve someone who runs off with someone else after five days of no phone calls. But then again, why am I feeling guilty?

KB hasn't even officially asked me to be his girlfriend. I don't dictate who he spends his evenings with or who he invites to dinner. Two of his previous girlfriends tried to march him to the altar, and at least he knows I won't do that if I'm out meeting other potential soulmates. How can you cheat on someone with whom you have no agreement? A harmless dinner can be just that, harmless – making friends before you even think about getting physical, although didn't I try that before?

To stay true to myself and my theories, I need to keep checking what else is out there before settling – although KB and I may be a while from that yet. I'm still convinced it's foolish to be faithful without an official commitment, but I don't want to keep wondering what I could be missing or if this is going to be for ever. I just want to be sure, for once.

In any case I sent KB a brief text as I was going home, having found two more missed calls from him and a rather sweet text. I wrote, 'I don't expect you to realise how upset I was at not hearing from you all week.'

I finally calmed down enough to return his calls this afternoon and he rang me back immediately. I really didn't know what to say. His explanation sounded plausible but crap: he left his charger at home. He couldn't get my number from his phone. He couldn't find a mobile phone shop or an internet café in the deeply rural place he was stuck in.

He apologised over and over, and asked me out to Italy 'next time'. He told me all about his trip and listened to my tales of sickness and work stress and everything else he'd missed out on.

But he didn't say anything about meeting up this weekend.

So I have made other plans. Sort of. I'm going out with Nicola tonight and hope to be busy tomorrow too. Not sure if he plans to do any more grovelling but he has to come up with *something* to make up for it.

Monday 12th March

In a nutshell, KB and I made up.

In a slightly larger nutshell – say, a coconut – with a bit more detail? He bought me lunch and we went to Hyde Park with two soft (cashmere?) blankets and a bottle of bubbly and cuddled and laughed till the sun went down. I told him about Random Bloke and he said that under the circumstances, he wouldn't have blamed me if I'd even slept with him after last week.

As we watched the sunset things turned slightly more naughty. He slipped his hand under my dress beneath the blanket and stroked me through my knickers. Then he pulled them aside and slipped a finger into my slickness. 'You are always wet when you're with me' – one of his most repeated observations. I couldn't return the favour because people were milling around and it would have been obvious what we were up to. And my hands were freezing, which probably wouldn't have helped matters.

He kept pushing his finger in and out of me, kissing me deeply and I played with my clit and lay back, blissed out till I came, looking up at the darkening sky through the tree branches above me.

We were getting cold by then (I wasn't wearing any stockings) so we packed up the remains of the liquid picnic and walked hand in hand through the dusky park until we found a taxi outside the gate.

He cooked me dinner back at his flat while I warmed up on the sofa, then we retreated to the bedroom. *My Big Fat Greek Wedding* was on TV and we settled on the bed. I lay close to him and began stroking his cock, until he told me in a low voice to put it in my mouth. He became rigid from my licking and

sucking, which turned me on even more. He began manoeu-
vring me on top of him and slipped inside me before I was
properly wet, but the slight friction made him feel amazing and
I rode astride him for a while. I actually nearly came without
even touching my clit, which is so rare for me I'd thought it
was a myth. Then my legs began to tire and I wanted him to
pause to put a condom on, so I switched to all fours but he
entered me from behind straight away.

What can I say? 'The heat of the moment'? We just 'got
carried away'? At one point I told him to 'come on my arse',
sure he'd pull out in time, but he must have thought that was
cancelled out by my encouraging 'don't stop, don't stop' and I
suddenly felt him coming inside me, and for a split second I felt
totally turned on and fulfilled.

Then it hit me.

'That was a mistake,' I told him as I rolled over to cuddle
him, 'I can't believe you came then. I think I'm ovulating.'

He should have known. It's not a good idea to sleep with a
woman who's so hormone driven she can't think straight, and
admits to being broody as hell. He's aware of my cycle but
chose to ignore it. I encouraged him to be stupid and he took
me up on it. We are both clean and healthy, haven't slept
around and love being close and naked together and I guess his
controlled and sympathetic reaction to our last 'crisis' encouraged me to throw caution to the wind and risk getting knocked
up by a guy I've only known for five months. He *does* keep
telling me he's older than his years, and not to worry. He *did*
volunteer the idea that he could cope with an unplanned child,
financially and emotionally.

He feels so fucking amazing inside me and I love the sensation of giving over all control to him, but now I'm in control.
And I don't like it. I'd rather not be in this situation. I'd rather

be with a loving, long-term partner in a stable, established relationship where I can look forward to what might happen when I sleep with him on the day I ovulate.

I asked KB when he thinks he'd be ready for kids.

'Thirty onwards,' he told me, so that's three years. I'll be thirty-three.

I don't want to wait that long. I can't.

I don't want to lose him either. I don't want to be a baby-crazed hormonal loony. I want to stop worrying that my tubes will stop working past thirty. I don't want to bring up a child on my own. I don't want the morning-bloody-after pill because I hate throwing up. I hate knowing that it prevents a fertilised egg from implanting in the womb.

What else do I hate? The thought of it *not* working. The anguish and the stress. Finding myself in a not-quite-relationship with possibly the most amazing guy I have met in three years and forcing decisions on him that are premature, to say the least.

I wish I had got more sleep last night.

I am glad I can talk to him about all this, because no one else understands. And he is very very sorry for having put me in this position.

Tuesday 13th March

As the morning-after pill goes to work on my unfertilised egg or stops a fertilised egg from implanting, I wonder if I was being too honest, telling KB what time of the month it was and actually going through with swallowing the damn thing.

Truth is, I'm shit scared of the consequences.

The Sailor texted me, en route to Canada. He said he'd spent the last few months sailing around some tropical islands, lucky bastard. We had a silly disagreement over the phone a while back and didn't speak for a long time, until last night. We still have that easy lover-friendship where we can tell each other anything, yet there's an undeniable spark. It wouldn't interfere if either of us were in a committed relationship though.

He's a fellow broody person too, so I texted him my dilemma.

Me: 'I'm still broody, but dating a twenty-seven year old.'

Him: 'What's annoying about a twenty-seven year old? Was seeing a Canadian girl during my trip and she may join me in Canada. Not sure.'

Me: 'Well, he's really great but not ready for kids. Canadians are great, good luck!' (I thought of Canada Boy and Blondie.)

Him: 'Cheers, but Canadian has no sense of humour, sadly. She does want kids though so I may have to compromise.'

Me: 'Awful to have to compromise. I have witty company but also the morning-after pill. Circumstances aren't always ideal.'

Him: 'LOL. I hear you. Hope it works out for you. Sometimes we have to compromise our ideals. As we get older they get harder to realise.'

Maybe, but it's hard to let them go . . .

Wednesday 14th March

I wonder if KB and I even speak the same language.

She says, 'I think you are too young for me, we may want different things.'

He says, 'How can you say that? I'm very mature.'

She thinks, great, he can imagine settling down and starting a family soon!

He says, 'I don't want to be an old dad.'

She thinks, he means over thirty.

He actually means over fifty.

He says, 'No matter what happens I will stick by you and support you.'

She thinks, how lovely, he wants a child with me.

He says, 'If we carry on like this, chances are something will happen sooner or later.'

She thinks, he'll be more careful from now on. If not, that means he doesn't mind the consequences.

Then he fucks up again and expects her to save his ass by swallowing a hormone bomb.

They go the theatre, then the pub, she gets drunk and sentimental, he drives her home.

He says, 'I want you to have what you want. I may not be the right guy for you. I am sorry for misleading you, I don't want to string you along. Maybe you should see other people. There is no way I can marry you within the year.'

She gets the message.

Friday 16th March

We haven't split – how could we if we were never together, at least as far as my theory goes? We're still 'seeing each other', which apparently involves a trip up north for the weekend to meet his folks. So I just got back from work and spent a few hours getting organised and primped and I'm waiting for KB to pick me up with his rusty, um, trusty steed and whisk me off into the sunset, or the night, at this rate.

Does it count as a dirty weekend if it involves staying in a flat overloaded with heirlooms and 'meeting the folks' is the first point on the agenda? I did shave my pussy with KB's razor this morning, seeing as he'd handily left it in my bathroom. It worked a treat – my lips are all creamy soft and velvety smooth. I only hope I didn't blunt his blade in the process, although he will reap the benefits.

Monday 19th March

KB is texting me as I type this, all sorry and guilty, lost and sad: 'I can't give you what you want and I don't want to keep stringing you along.'

The fissure that opened up last week got wider over our dirty weekend. It didn't get off to a great start.

After a very nasty near-accident a few years back where I spun a car containing my family in sleet and snow at 100 mph, I'm something of a nervous passenger. Driving in rain and darkness makes it worse. As we were heading up the motorway the car in front braked sharply and I yelped, seeing us crashing into it and spinning off the road, and KB retorted rather sharply, 'I don't need a backseat driver. That car wasn't even braking.' How could I tell that when the rain was streaking the windscreen, not exactly helped by his dodgy wiper blades?

When we got to the flat the first thing staring me in the face was another edition of that framed photo of him and his ex. So she's been here too? Great. I went to the loo and when I came back he'd turned it flat on its face. We were both tired and decided to unwind by drinking too much whisky, and cuddling. We fell into bed, and he made me come with his tongue then with his dick inside me, and then I stroked and sucked him to orgasm before we fell asleep.

In the morning we made love again, with him being especially careful to make it 'safe' (albeit in the wrong half of my cycle) and taking ages to come. He suggested some bargain hunting at the local outlet shopping centre, then when I was trying to shop myself to oblivion to distract myself from the bad feeling churning inside me he got impatient. I spotted Calvin Klein bras for £2 each and left him with my bags while I disappeared into the changing rooms, thinking there wasn't a problem because he'd assured me he was 'fine' and I took him at his word. After all, he'd wanted to shop. When I emerged he looked stony, and complained about a cold coming on, and that 'we won't have much time in town'.

So why didn't he just drag me away? My attempts to turn it into a joke misfired, and it was difficult to stay cheerful enough to stop him strangling me with my new underwear. We left, only to realise we had loads of time to kill before meeting his mum, so he took me to the top of a department store where there was a beautiful view of a church and I bought a bottle of champagne for later.

I wanted to look nice for tea with the folks, and planned to get changed in the car which we'd parked down a quiet street, but fastening the stockings to my suspender belt in the cramped space of a car which was slowly beginning to steam up proved more difficult than I had anticipated. Unable to help (I don't think they teach boys how to snap suspender buttons at public school) while I got more and more flustered, KB just had to sit and wait, glaring at his watch in frustration.

'I find this hard to handle, constantly being late and disorganised,' he told me when I asked what the matter was. I apologised and tried to make light of it, but when I rolled up the second stocking I laddered it with my watch strap in the process. I burst into laughter, which, thank God, he joined me in. I took the stockings off and we weren't late at all, which made his criticism feel a bit unfair to say the least.

Dinner was lovely. I was decidedly overdressed for fish and

chips, but got on well with his mum and stepdad, whose accents were nowhere near as posh as his.

When we walked back to the apartment I suggested going to a pub for St Patrick's Day, but he refused. 'People like me get beaten up in places like that,' was his excuse, implying that everyone was chavvy and provincial. I tore him off a strip for being a snob. I'd been out in that town before, and everyone had been friendly, even when I won the karaoke competition. So what was his problem? Maybe the pub we went past doesn't usually attract a crowd of overweight toffs, but I could hardly see him getting a black eye for wearing a cashmere jumper. We stayed in and drank all the champagne, followed by some whisky. There was nothing on TV. He refused sex. We cuddled and fell asleep naked.

On Sunday I woke up hungover and began gently stroking his nipple without much thought. After a little while he looked at me intensely, rolling over to meet my gaze, then kissed me deeply. 'What's that?' I asked him, 'What are you planning to do?' 'I want to screw you,' he replied, and moved his hand down to my crotch. 'You are always wet,' he said as he stroked me slowly.

'What if I don't let you?' I wanted to know. 'Would you try and screw me anyway?'

'Yes, I would pull your hair and hold you down and fuck you hard,' he pushed a finger inside me and placed my hand on his hard dick. I was pleasantly surprised to find him so turned on. My body tingled in anticipation of what he'd do to me, and he pushed my legs apart, rolled on a condom and entered me slowly.

I think this was the first time I saw him properly in unforgiving daylight, close up and naked, and I surprised myself with how much I still wanted him and to fuck him although he looked like a fat, dishevelled ogre. Albeit one with the most beautiful eyes in the world.

He rolled on top of me, pushing me down and putting his full weight on me, like I'd wanted him to do for weeks, and I pulled him right into me, although it hurt a little, because I needed him and for everything to be all right again. He held my wrist and I grabbed his hair, he grabbed my hair and I scratched his back, pulling him deeper into me, then I turned over to ride him with his balls between my legs.

I came with a yell and he kept on pounding me. I felt absolutely amazing and we screwed on the rickety bed until my legs started to hurt. He refused to fuck me from behind, saying he liked me just where he had me, and his eyes had a lusty, loved-up glaze. He took the condom off and stroked himself as I pretended to hold him down, then took a sip of water and took his cock in my mouth. He moaned and I thought he'd come right there and then, then I sucked the water down and gulped on his dick as he went on wanking. 'This was all the way inside you,' he told me, 'fucking you.' I sat back and watched as he stroked himself, leaning down to lick him occasionally and wrapping my hair round his balls, then he pushed my head away and came on his stomach with a groan. I put his dick back in my mouth after he spilled the last drop, sucking him and massaging the sensitive spot between his legs. 'This feels amazing,' he whispered.

He never mentioned that the night before, three-quarters of the way down the bottle of champagne, I'd told him I loved him. I hope he was so drunk he forgot. I bet he hopes I was too drunk to remember.

I miss our fun times, the carefree way I used to feel about him, even if I was nursing the secret thought of how perfect he would be as the father of my children. Yes, he's trying to 'do the decent thing' now by holding back and not stringing me along, but that makes me love him more. And yes, I did say love.

I felt like crying the whole time.

Monday 26th March

I went round to KB's flat at midnight last night. I couldn't stand the distance and coldness that had suddenly come up between us and I was scared to lose him without a last chance to talk face to face. Even though I woke him he told me it was sweet of me to turn up.

We chatted for ages downstairs in the hall and he just looked so sad and empty. He thinks he isn't the right man for me because his life plan is so different from mine, and nothing I said would convince him otherwise. He was a little stand-offish but then let me cuddle him and I felt a bit closer even though the light in his eyes had gone out.

I could see that he has taken everything I said to him so much to heart and it has hurt him deeply. He feels guilty for 'misleading' me – something I never accused him of – and for not taking the opportunities to tell me we weren't heading the same way. I wanted him to understand that I wasn't trying to get pregnant by him, but I wouldn't mind it if it had happened by accident. I agree we have to spend more time together and get to know each other, but the B.A.B.Y. subject was pushed up to the surface so soon that now it's hard to ignore it and carry on as if nothing's been said.

'I wish I had kept my mouth shut,' I told him, expecting the tears to come but my eyes stayed dry. He doesn't agree, thinks it's important to get things out in the open and talk, but I feel like I'm being punished.

He let me stay and we cuddled and fell asleep, in that oddly asexual way.

In the morning he walked me to the tube and we hugged goodbye. My last words to him were that I'd give him time and wait for *him* to get in touch.

9

Office Romance

SPRING/SUMMER 2007

Thursday 29th March

I don't know what to write because I don't know what to think.

KB called last night just when I was trying to drink myself into oblivion on free cocktails. I don't know what he wanted, really. We had a brief chat, me on the staircase of the club, him at Piccadilly Circus, about the same thing, over and over. I tried to sound upbeat. Well, I guess I was upbeat. No, I was just trying to be.

Really I am just sad. And I feel rejected. He kept going, 'I'm sorry, I'm sorry.'

He thinks it's all just hopeless now. Whatever. I told him not to call me today as I had a date (I do, but it's probably a bad idea to rush out and do this when I'm so emotionally raw). But what's the alternative? Lying on my sofa and crying? Answering Rugby Boy's texts? Calling one of my unsympathetic friends? By the time I cycled home last night I was so drunk that I don't know how I managed it. I seem to have stopped wearing my helmet too. Not a good combination of circumstances, but at least I should burn off some of those cocktail and canapés, and all those breakfasts so beautifully cooked by KB.

Tuesday 3rd April

I think I've been too depressed to write. I mean, what else is there to say? KB came over on Sunday. We'd both been down and wanted to see each other, but I suspect for rather different reasons. He didn't bring flowers, chocolates or a cuddly toy. He brought a pregnancy test so we could be reassured that the morning-after pill had worked. Nice.

I packed some chilled bubbly and we went to the park but it wasn't a revival of our romp under the picnic blankets, just a post mortem tinged with extra sadness. As the champagne began to take effect it came spilling out of my eyes as I realised that even though he hadn't said it in so many words, it was over.

Why would I want to keep seeing him 'as a friend'? Maybe in a few months' time, but now, no contact is the only thing I can do. He thinks I am taking it too personally. Then he said, 'These past two weeks have been the most down I've been in my entire life,' which was possibly an exaggeration because he followed it with, 'I just don't think it could work between us because I couldn't live with you.'

My stomach seized up. I'd tried to be all fun, light and lovely, I'd made an effort with a cute skirt, low-cut top and lacy leggings, and he says this?

I can't tell you how insulted I was. *He* can't live with *me*?

At least I hoover my fucking floor. I flush the toilet and my feet don't smell, nor do I take three hours to come or look fat naked. My flat isn't freezing. My fridge is clean.

As I sat there seething he said, 'You get so frustrated and angry sometimes and I don't like conflict.' What if I had a good reason to be angry? Oh, apparently I have no good reasons to be angry. Right. Maybe I'm not allowed to be angry or depressed.

I used to like his calm, his measured, kind way of reassuring me. No more, I fear. No more. I mustn't forget that he *cares*, *oh so much*.

Thursday 5th April

To top it all, my new lodger has to move out because his job is so poorly paid. I told him a new job would be easier to find than a new cheap flat. You live and learn. The next one had better have a payslip handy for me to check out . . .

At work Tall Boy breezed in, just back from his umpteenth holiday this year. I was curious to find out how he'd liked South America, but he was more interested in finding out how I'd been: 'So, what have you been up to?' 'Oh, getting dumped.' I didn't want to go into details with everyone else around, but he was immediately sympathetic. 'You said he was too young for you. I couldn't believe he was only twenty-seven. I thought he was at least forty.' 'Well, he dresses older,' I agreed.

Straight away he suggested we go out for drinks soon. I am tempted to arrange something for Friday thirteenth, my lucky day.

Easter Sunday 8th April

Today saw me battling along a windy, sunny beach, pushing a buggy. Two posh boys with a rugby ball walked by, struggling to chuck it between them against the breeze. One was wearing trendy aviator sunglasses with a gold rim, the other a white pair, and they looked relaxed, handsome and very young. Not surprising in a student town.

'It won't happen,' I shouted against the howl of the wind, 'the wind is too strong – I tried earlier,' and my smile indicated the toddler's warm, sleeping form in the buggy and the neon green football on the rack beneath. I'd been running after a man all weekend, or at least, his ball – against the wind, down slopes and into thorny bushes. But oh, it was much more fun than chasing after grown-up men with their stupid commitment issues!

I felt relaxed, fulfilled and rewarded, even if nothing much was happening to saturate my day with excitement. His screams and occasional tantrums saw me reaching for tissues, the spoon, his nappy-clad bottom, and sorting the problem. He calmed down as easily as he got excited, and I was rewarded by slobbery kisses, a constantly runny nose, soft, soft skin to graze against my cheek, downy hair, and laughter that tickled the bottom of my soul.

Nothing I couldn't handle, even if the day and the hours stretched – there was always another beach to explore, a café to sit in, a kite to watch, ducks to feed, ice cream to buy and a nice comfy home to go back to. I knew it was for a short time only and his parents would be there to take him from me as soon as I got back to the house, grateful and with food and smiles waiting for me.

I wouldn't abduct him, I reassured his mum, I'd rather make my own, but his presence in my arms quietened my soul. I felt loved and useful, even if only for wielding tissues and fetching balls. 'He suits you,' she smiled, watching me with the pram.

In the evening I turned him over to his parents. They aren't married but their relationship has spanned twelve years and two continents. I have trouble binding someone to me for three months, even when I've adopted his city as my own for years now. I'm glad I left London for some peace and some fresh sea air.

Monday 9th April

Thursday night me and two friends visiting from home ended up at the Easter party in Boujis, where bunny girls were handing out chocolate vodka shots by the gallon. Somehow six of those shots found their way into my mouth, and that same mouth then asked one of the roaming massage girls swanning about the place for what turned out to be easily the best massage I'd had all year.

I kissed some guy I'd barely met and the next morning he was on the phone, eager to arrange a date, but trouble is, I don't know if I can be bothered. He's keen on sailing. Yacht Boy.

Rugby Boy has been on my case for weeks, wanting to meet up when he returns from skiing. Tall Boy might be mine for the taking when we have that drink he's suddenly so keen on. The Sailor wants to meet up for lunch. Someone from that ad I posted late last year (the one that netted me KB) has been badgering me too.

How come you only want what you can't have? There's candy everywhere, the boy equivalent of chocolate vodka shots, but I don't want any. I don't fancy going through the motions of 'the first few months' with somebody new. I have no desire to call any of them or to hold my breath in anticipation of their calls.

I miss the sex, I miss KB and our conversations and he's ignoring me. I know he doesn't want to be with me, but I refuse to accept that I'm worthless to him, that it meant nothing and that I could easily find someone who moves me like he did again.

I know he's not my ideal man, but if it hurts this much to be rejected by someone who's – I don't know – 70 per cent right, what would it feel like to lose someone who's 100 per cent right?

I want to put my head in the sand, under the duvet, under water in the bath and stop breathing for a while. Just stop thinking.

Sweet Ex called and I confessed that I'd been dumped because many guys don't realise that women come with a sell-by date. 'That's so sad,' he said, 'a sell-by date.'

And he meant it in the sense of 'regrettable', not 'pathetic'.

Saturday 14th April

I can't believe I slept with Tall Boy last night.

I mean, that was my dream come true. I've fancied the pants off him since October and it was wonderful, better than I could have hoped. He made love to me like I'd like to make love for the rest of my life. Then he left without so much as a cup of coffee this morning.

I've been hanging around at home with a hangover and a confused head all day, despite the glorious weather. I feel stupid, used, angry at myself for getting drunk, inviting him back and then inviting him to stay the night.

Angry because I didn't set a framework for this encounter, it all just happened in the heat of the moment. I didn't stop him. I'm proud, too, to have finally gotten him into bed, fulfilled by the memory of his stubble on my pussy, his tongue on my clit, his finger inside me, my vagina swelling at his thrusts, tightening as he pumped into me. It was so intense that when he came I burst into tears, although I managed to hide it well I think.

I have never felt anything like it.

I'd taken him out with a bunch of friends and we'd gone to the club with the secret room again, which I just had to show to Tall Boy. When we rejoined the others, things had changed between us. We suddenly had this incredible chemistry, and every time we could snatch a kiss without everyone seeing, we couldn't keep our hands and lips off one another. One thing, as they say, led to another.

The tip of his penis was the smoothest I have ever tasted; he was hard as a rocket, the perfect body . . . Not too slight, not fat, the perfect weight on me. His orgasm was the most amazing I've ever experienced. I literally felt my vagina stretch even more when his cum pumped into the condom and we stayed locked together while he caught his breath and my shivers subsided.

I don't know if this was a one-off and I feel ashamed that I didn't wait until things between us were clearer. He probably sees this as an ultra-casual thing. After all, he knows I just split up from KB and he hasn't given any indication about whether this meant anything to him or if we're going to do it again in the future. I wish sex wouldn't leave me feeling so vulnerable.

I'm realising again that each time my pussy gets some action my heart appears to want to get in on it too. I mean, if you have sex with someone you like but you're not sure they like you back, you are bound to feel a bit insecure. This multi-dating seems to mean I'm forever at the 'does he like me?' stage, pretending that I don't care about the answer. After being so close to KB I'm starting to hanker for something more, but how do I have a real relationship without going through this again? It's impossible.

I am stupid, stupid, stupid. Why not play hard to get for a change? Or stop after a second cocktail? Why couldn't I find the moment to tell him I couldn't do this just now and I needed to clear my head first? And now all I can think of is that he was so keen to get out of my flat this morning that he turned down coffee and a shower, and just gave me a quick kiss on the lips.

When I think about seeing him at work I am overwhelmed by a sense of doom. This is so screwed up. I have to see it as just a nice night, a chance to validate my attractiveness and, maybe, something to do again, soon. But mainly I feel cheap and confused and want to punch someone.

And six paracetamol haven't stopped this headache.

Monday 16th April

You know what? Sitting here at work I'm thinking I should be proud I got that sexy man into bed. I saw him lick my juice off his fingers and heard him tell me he likes the smell of my breath, the way I kiss and my fingers on his cock. So why should I care if he didn't want to try my coffee?

He's not due to work here for a week or so. We'll see.

Tuesday 17th April

For sale by auction: one key.

To a little apartment in Kensington, consisting of a lounge/kitchen, a double bedroom which functions as a walk-in wardrobe, and an en-suite bathroom.

Floors throughout are covered with crumbs and bits of wrapping foil, the toilet is plumbically challenged and won't flush properly, hence you need a good air freshener, an iron bladder and a tolerant nose.

The fridge is permanently overfilled and the freezer compartment hasn't been defrosted in years, but there is plenty of storage for foie gras and champagne. The apartment is freezing in winter due to draughty windows and you'd need to be more generous or wealthy than its current occupant to heat it properly. Peeling wallpaper and rickety curtain rails included.

The panoramic view into neighbouring multi-million-pound apartments which have been modernised or at least decorated in the last decade make this bachelor pad a real gem.

Do not bid if allergic to dust, due to the large volume of antique books piled up everywhere. Send your highest bid in strictest confidence to the author of this blog.

Lost: rose-tinted spectacles.

If found, please return to yours truly. I can't see without them.

Finder's fee: a cashmere hat and a designer bag, no longer needed due to attached memories.

Thursday 19th April

Up at two-twenty a. m. this morning.

I was leafing through a book, trying to go back to sleep, when I saw the word 'Kensington' and found my body shaking in a slow sob which led to crying full tilt. I rang his number twice and let it ring, number withheld. No answer. Then I got a pair of scissors and chopped up the cashmere socks he left behind. I put the fluffy pieces in the bin, but I couldn't stop crying.

I dialled Canada Boy's number in Toronto, desperate to speak to someone who wouldn't strangle me because of the time. He answered and I could hear people in the background.

'It's Sienna,' I sobbed and sniffed.

'Sienna, man, what's up?'

And I realised how much I missed him. Our easy, non-judgemental, spontaneous, honest and close friendship. Every time I saw him we just had such a blast.

'I can't stop crying,' I told him. He knows all about KB, having had his two cents' worth in an MSN chat the other night, but he was confused.

'Is this about a new guy?' he asked, and to be honest I can understand the confusion. After all, didn't I tell him we broke up a month ago?

He managed to calm me down and, curled under the duvet, cradling the handset, I blurted out that I had found it so hard to get close to anyone for such a long time because of Pinocchio, and that that was why I hadn't let him get close to me, and how last time I attempted to see someone without immediately sleeping with them, they dumped me after a few months. Remember the Nice Guy whom I was seeing after the split with Pinocchio, before I had my fateful chat about multi-dating with Canada Boy? He got fed up when I still wouldn't come home with him after two months and stopped calling me, so it's best not to risk it. I can't win.

I feel like I'm running out of ways to assess a guy's true intentions. Englishmen never want to be 'just friends' before taking things further.

Canada told me all the right things, that I was young, gorgeous, talented, I'd meet the right guy, it was his loss, etc., etc., . . . I started to feel a little better but felt guilty for keeping Canada from his guests so we chatted about mutual friends and his plans to come to London soon, then rang off.

I think if I got involved with someone I really cared about, I wouldn't be able to deal with the break-up. Actually I know I wouldn't cope, because I lost the plot so completely when I discovered Pinocchio's continued involvement with his ex.

Immediately after we split I had to go on a work trip that left me stewing, sleepless in a hotel in another town for five nights and only just making it through my meetings during the days. By the Saturday when I tried to go over to his flat to collect my stuff I wasn't exactly myself – let's put it that way.

Maybe if he hadn't double-locked the door because he

thought I'd boil his cat (as if! I loved that cat – still do), I wouldn't have been so frustrated that I was unable to pick up my stuff whilst he was out. Maybe if I'd slept a bit or he'd been there to talk to me I wouldn't have felt so angry. Maybe if I hadn't tried an alternative way in and discovered there wasn't one, but found myself under his floorboards with no way into the flat, I wouldn't have felt so powerless. Maybe if there hadn't been a supermarket with squid and raw chicken on special offer, maybe *maybe*, I wouldn't have found myself crawling under his bedroom in my pink suede boots, using the torch on my mobile phone to find a spot to mix up a special treat of seafood, poultry, yeast and milk that was gonna be a gift to him that went on giving. Maybe.

But I did mean to tell him about it. I really did.

And the thing is, even that didn't improve my state of mind. I think I normally keep that bit of my brain locked up in a padded cell, but that day it was out and rampaging around and everything I did, I did on impulse. I can't say I had it planned. A few hours after I'd hauled myself out of the improvised trap door, Samantha phoned to say that Pinocchio had told her he'd unlocked the door and I could go and get my stuff as long as she was there to 'supervise'.

Only Sam didn't bother to turn up.

And so there I was in the flat which had felt like home for the best part of a year, cooking him special dinners and giving him back massages in the bath. I couldn't cry any more. I wanted him to really see how much he'd upset me with his lies.

I took:

* The shower head (I paid for it, after all).
* A lamp I bought him.
* The bedspread I gave him to keep the cat hair out of the sheets.

- My sister's book that he'd been reading.
- A picture frame with lots of pictures of us – a Valentine's present from me.

I left:

- Some boots which were uncomfortable.
- A clothes dummy which I put under the sheets in his bed to freak him out.
- Photos of us stuck to the fridge.
- A nightie.

I destroyed:

- His bitch's mug.
- Her photographs and some paperwork he'd been looking after for her.
- A card she sent him.

Then I:

- Poured her perfume down the loo.
- Peed in the perfume bottle and replaced the cap.
- Tipped all the red wine down the loo and left it unflushed.
- Hid all her expensive books in the shed.
- Took all her shoes and clothes and bagged them for the local charity shop.
- Stopped to fuss the cat, who'd been watching all this, and say goodbye.
- Dropped the keys through the letter box.

Like I said, I wasn't exactly myself.
But at least I didn't:

- Empty the stinky kitty litter in his bed.
- Write a letter to his mum telling her about his drug habit and his exes' abortions.
- Shit in his fridge.
- Wee in his expensive whisky.
- Post his number as a free gay taxi service.
- Call the people he owes money and give them his work address.
- Shag his best friend.
- Park his car at a bus stop.

In retrospect, it should have been a massive clue to me that so many of her things were still in the flat she'd supposedly moved out of a year before, and it was only due to my extreme tolerance or naivety that I didn't question why a man would keep looking after his ex's stuff indefinitely, and put her up in his flat every time she chose to visit London.

After I'd dropped off the bag of clothes at Oxfam, I suddenly felt like all the anger drained right out of me and there was nothing but sadness left in my stomach. What had happened to me? I sat down on the pavement with my head in my hands and stared at my feet without seeing them, trying to breathe deeply and fight the panic that was welling up.

What had I done? And why had I done it when all I wanted was to talk to Pinocchio and have some answers? Why did he tell me he wanted to marry me if he was still in love with her? Did he ever mean it? What was I supposed to do now? Why did I miss him so much it hurt? Would he apologise, give me the hug I badly needed? Reassure me?

After a while, someone came out of a shop to ask if I was OK, and I thanked them and got up a little shakily. I took myself to my doctor's surgery where my GP took one look at me and promised to give me priority on the waiting list for counselling. I limped off home and dived into bed with my clothes on, praying for sleep.

Oh, and Pinocchio moved out of that flat a few weeks later, oddly enough.

Monday 23rd April

Tall Boy is coming to the office tomorrow, wahey! New project – he's coming in for an initial meeting with my boss and to do some sketches. I admit I'm a bit nervous and a bit peeved that he hasn't been in touch, so yeah, maybe I feel a bit used. But also a bit horny. Actually, more than a bit horny, as he's been the object of my wanking fantasies for these past two weeks.

I just can't get the smooth taste of his cock in my mouth out of my head, and I want him in my pussy again.

Wednesday 25th April

With a spring in my step, a swing in my hips, a twinkle in my eyes and a misting of dew in my knickers I came to work yesterday, knowing he'd be back.

Every time my boss was out of the room we stole kisses. When the boss was fiddling with the photocopier, Tall Boy sent me an MSN: 'I am trying to sort out these new designs . . . but I'd rather do it with my cock in your mouth.'

He lured me out to lunch, holding my hand as soon as we were out of sight of the office. 'A proper date,' I joked, when he paid. 'A date at lunchtime for people with busy lives,' he laughed, and we snogged frantically before strolling back, and he pushed me into a doorway and put my hand on his crotch so I could feel how hard he was.

'Fuck me, fuck me!' my pussy whispered, moistening in anticipation.

'Take me, take me!' shivered my body when his hands gripped me hard.

'Love me, love me!' pleaded my eyes, my lips on his stubble, my fingers in his soft curly hair. So I closed them.

And meanwhile, my brain was silently screaming, 'What the fuck is going on? First you couldn't even get him to go for a cocktail with you, then he was 'too respectful' of your relationship with KB, now he won't let go of your tongue or your hand or your booty. What are you? A toy?'

At our desks, I snuck over for a kiss and a grope and he was still hard. 'Shame that desk doesn't have a long table cloth,' I teased him. 'You could tell my boss: "Oh, Sienna's just popped out to the shops."' I got a wicked grin in return.

'Do you still speak to KB?' he wanted to know later. This seemed like a caring thing to ask but because I didn't really want to go into it we touched briefly on his ex before moving onto a different subject.

Was he trying to find out if I was definitely available now? I took it as a good sign that he's interested in me.

At the end of the day he kissed me on the lips and said, 'See you soon,' and that was it. My feelings are all over the shop and my pussy is lonely and confused.

At least I have the satisfaction of knowing he went home with seriously blue balls.

Wednesday 2nd May

Tall Boy is starting to get on my nerves. Who'd have thought it? His MSN conversation is tantamount to sexual harassment – all about how he's planning a visit to the office, and 'maybe we'll get to use that empty room upstairs' and 'will your boss be in?', but when I try and half jokingly, half seriously, ask him what the hell is going on, he just avoids the question. Or else leads me a merry dance. Let me show you:

Sienna: 'You like things to progress at a steady pace, don't you? First, months of no interest, suddenly it's hard cocks at dawn!'

Tall Boy: 'Haha, yes indeed. Hard cocks at the crack of dawn.'

Sienna: 'Seriously, I thought this was a one-nighter after your swift exit . . .'

Tall Boy: 'No chance.'

Sienna: 'Chance? Would be a fine thing.'

Tall Boy: 'The thought of you sucking me off has made me ridiculously horny.'

Sienna: 'Listen buster, you gotta make up your mind about me.'

Tall Boy: 'Huh?'

Sienna: 'I dunno, usually it takes people a while to get to that full-on sex talk. And they tend to speak about other things too!'

Tall Boy: 'Did I mention that I'd like to rub your tits while your legs are wrapped round my shoulders? Then after a nice long fuck, cum all over them?'

Sienna: 'Ahhhhhhhhhhhh!'

Thursday 3rd May

It's just struck me that Tall Boy is incredibly stupid.

1. He missed the signs I was giving him for months and months.

2. He slept with me when I was drunk. It's never that good when she's drunk, boys, and can lead to all sorts of complications.

3. He's just started something that can only be described as a sordid affair with me, the person who works for one of his employers. And who could see to it that his company loses our business. Maybe it would be smarter if he actually thought ahead and at least gave me the illusion that he cares?

He's not alone, though. I, too, am incredibly stupid. I'm the one who sent him a text late last night saying, 'You've got me thinking about your hard cock.'

'What a pity,' he texted back, 'that you weren't thinking about it an hour ago. I was on the tube and could have made a little stop to show it to you. Sweet dreams xx'

This takes the prize for stupid. Just fucking ring the girl, ring her bell and fuck her senseless. She's so stupid she'd probably do it.

Tuesday 8th May

Captain Letdown strikes again.

Tall Boy told me he'd be in the office today, so I put on a short skirt (despite the wind), and even did my make-up this morning. Here I am, looking cute and there's no one here to appreciate it. Not that I'd let him do anything more than admire me from a distance – seeing as all he wants is a no-strings affair to brighten up his week.

Friday 11th May

'Let me show you some outlines,' he said, beckoning me over to the desk.

I approached and was confronted by the image of a glossy, shaved, nude-apart-from-a-red-belt woman making love to two headless men. One had his ass facing her, his cock in her willing pussy (yes, that's still confusing me too), the other one hung somewhat unenthusiastically into her mouth. At least he was wearing a wedding ring. So the guy in her cunt was the best man? I burst out laughing and returned to my desk.

'Do you have a lot of porn on your computer?' I asked him.

'Oh, this is just something my friend sent me,' he said. Yeah, right.

Last week's foul mood has lifted. A few things happened:

+ A second illicit lunch with our graphic designer.
+ His sweet text last night.
+ His lips, his hair, his kisses.
+ The arrival of my period (must every month be a pregnancy scare? Even after that well-timed helping of Levonelle?)
+ The absolute knowledge that I will have him again, on his turf, on my terms.
+ His laughter, his smell, his energy.
+ How shy he seemed in person after all that cocky MSN messaging.

The boss left us alone in the office, so we went to the kitchen to 'make tea' and ended up in one corner, his hand up my skirt, touching my clit lightly through my knickers, my hand caressing his stiff cock through his jeans, his delicious kisses deep in my mouth. Getting wet, moaning with pleasure . . .

I heard a noise from next door and stiffened; Tall Boy was back at his desk before you could say 'horny'. Later, when I was 'making tea' again, I put my hand inside his trousers, wanting to check if his dick really was as smooth as I'd remembered.

'I won't lick it,' I warned him as he started unbuttoning his flies. He breathed heavily and pressed his fingers hard against my clit. 'Why not?' he asked. 'At least then we can say we've done it in the office.' Oh, the logic of randy men!

So then I had to. I mean, I had to check if it tasted and felt as good as I remembered (chocolate connoisseurs call it the 'in-mouth feel') and I wanted to say I'd done it in the office too; oh, and because there were no other freelancers in to interrupt us.

I bent my knees slowly and sucked him into my mouth . . .

Thankfully my ears still work when I've got my mouth full, and the sound of my boss coming down the corridor – surprise! – alerted me. I jumped up, dropping his cock, and Tall Boy, eyes widening, quickly buttoned up his jeans. When my boss walked in he found me alone in the kitchen, innocently stirring two cups of tea while Tall Boy tapped away on his computer.

'Would you like a cup of tea?' I asked him as I washed my hands and wiped them on a dish cloth in the interest of hygiene. To my relief he declined. Just as well, I would have had the dumbest grin on my face when I served it.

I still don't know Tall Boy's plans for the weekend, let alone the rest of his life. And I don't know why all he apparently wants is a casual fling if all his mates are getting married.

Saturday 12th May

Why am I still obsessed with KB and even Cashmere and the reasons they left me and refused to keep in touch?

I was at a gig, surrounded by happy people, sipping on a great cocktail after just nearly beating a really cute guy at pool, when it hit me: I am on my own. KB has rejected me and I still lust after his green eyes, his chubby hands on my body, his wet dick on my thigh, his wit, his voice . . . So I dial his number.

Number withheld and it's too loud to hear anything anyway, but he picks up. I hang up and dial again. People around me are dancing and having fun, I should be making conversation with them or something.

This time KB speaks but I can't hear what he's saying. I'm sure he knows it's me. I know he doesn't have many mates, which makes his avoidance of me even more personal and painful. If we still spoke I'm sure I'd feel better about all this. He just doesn't want me. He doesn't want me.

And now champagne and charity shops and gentlemen's clubs and cashmere are always going to be tainted. And in an attempt to act out an alternative reality I keep buying myself fake engagement rings and obsessing over pregnancy tests.

I asked the boy I'd been playing pool with to explain something for me. Last week Yacht Boy – he of the Easter snog at Boujis – took me out for dinner then invited me to his parents' house in their absence for sailing. But then I didn't hear from him for a week. The cute boy was stumped: 'Women think too much. I dunno, maybe he's just not that into you? Or his parents came home unexpectedly?'

'Was it because I asked him if I'd have my own bedroom in their house?' I proffered. No useful answer was forthcoming. Or maybe Yacht Boy realised he was just a Band-Aid being used to fix an open sore, and that sex with the recently bereaved is not worth the can of worms it opens.

It was raining so I hung around a little before cycling home, then got soaked anyway. Tall Boy texted and asked if I'd come to Covent Garden. Too late. But at least he was thinking of me, or else just drunk.

Monday 14th May

My spies tell me Tall Boy was sighted having a good old laugh with two girls in a pub on Friday night. In a way I'm hurt – I thought after work he'd go home, have a shower and phone me, begging me to come over. Maybe he sensed that I would have told him no to preserve a smidgen of dignity and self-respect, although I would have been very tempted as I was already 'buttered up' by our afternoon's shenanigans. He's been quiet and I've been quiet apart from that text on Saturday, but according to my friend who spotted him, I should just enjoy the flirting at the office and the occasional free lunch. No word from Yacht Boy either. Do I trust these men? No. Do I love any of them? No. Are they making me feel great? No. Whatever . . .

Monday 28th May

Pinocchio and his new girlfriend are getting married some time this summer. I bet Sam is the bloody bridesmaid. Why do I care? Why indeed. Maybe because in the last two years all I've gotten is dumped (although I've had a lot of fun in the process, I should add), while he's slipping his debt-ridden ring onto her stinky finger. Good luck to them, I suppose.

Apparently Tall Boy didn't mean to treat me as a convenient

substitute for a brothel the other night when he texted from Covent Garden, instead he was taken aback to find out what I thought he had meant by 'coming over tonight' without offering so much as a pizza in return. Having been his colleague and friend for over six months I feel I deserve more than the classic booty text, I mean, what an insult! If he'd had an actual plan like a film or a dinner, or given me more notice I would have been flattered and may well have been up for any ensuing passion. But his casual, late-night request for my company felt an awful lot like he didn't much care either way and I think I'm worth more effort than that. He trailed off into an apologetic 'I just don't get women' speech. I could tell by his face and his reaction that he hadn't meant it like that at all, it was simply his clumsy way of showing he wanted to see me, so all was forgiven and we swiftly moved on to more fun things.

Neither of us was concentrating much on the figures on our screens, being totally absorbed by the figure at the desk opposite. When the other freelancer was in the kitchen making us coffee, he came over, stroked and kissed my neck and grabbed my back, and I felt myself slicken up in anticipation at the naughtiness of it all.

Kisses and cuddles, and lingering glances were exchanged frequently as we tried to catch up with our work load. And at one point I even chanced sitting on his lap for a deep, slow kiss, while our ears strained to hear my boss shifting next door.

When the boss finally left for a late lunch, leaving only Tall Boy, me and the freelancer in the office, things were reaching a pitch. I watched the digits changing on my computer clock, watched the freelancer stretch, look like she was about to go to lunch, then sit back down at her computer to check an email. Eventually she left, and Tall Boy and I barely looked at each other, but raced for the stairs. On the second floor of the building there's a room with a sofa in it which might be another office at some point, if the business expands. I hauled the blind down, leaving suspicious finger prints on the dusty wood frame, and turned to look at him.

Would we really go through with it? Would the boss catch us? Would Tall Boy respect me after this? I didn't care. I was too horny, and I knew that Tall wouldn't be working on this project with us for much longer. Opportunities would be thin on the ground in the future.

He sat back on the sofa and I straddled him, kissing him deeply and trying to peer into his green eyes – which he kept closed for some annoying reason – wondering if he was thinking of someone else. He pawed and groped me with his big hands to the point where it was almost painful, but very, very erotic nonetheless.

I can't have guys pussyfooting around me, with gentle tickling fingers and barely there touches. I want men to act like *men*, and crush me and fuck me hard because my curves make them feel out of control.

He unzipped his flies and his hard dick sprang out. I'd known all day long how turned on he was, but it was nice to see it for myself, and I lowered my lips around him and licked him gently, then sucked hungrily and he flung his head back and moaned. I grabbed his shirt and pulled him over on top of me, lying back with my legs spread and my mouth open for him to kiss. He unzipped my jeans and pushed my knickers aside and I slipped a hand down into my wetness, then offered him my fingers to lick eagerly before I sucked his dick once more.

My top was off, up over my head, and I was splayed on the sofa in my bra and knickers, Tall Boy was fiddling with a condom he'd pulled out of his trouser pocket and I knew I wanted, no, needed him to fuck me, but was sincerely hoping my boss would take as long over lunch as he usually did, and not remember that he and Tall Boy had an appointment in 20 minutes. I quickly pulled my top back on, just in case, and Tall Boy lowered himself between my legs, pushed my pants aside and entered me forcefully, raw and unstoppable, clasping my wrists above my head in his hands.

'Oh my God,' he breathed, and I knew he wasn't far off, but I wanted him to come and I wanted it to last for ages too, but the clock in my head was ticking and I knew we had to be fast.

A few forceful, determined strokes of his hard, thick cock later, I could tell he was holding back so he wouldn't explode. Christ, it had been over a month since the last time and this time I was sober and it was daylight and I wanted him so, so much. His smell, his weight on me, his voice, his breath, his cock inside me, the look in his eyes . . . I tried to make myself come with my hand while he pumped away slowly, then just told him to go for it, to fuck me hard, and he did, violently, affectionately and without regret.

He came within a few seconds and I held him inside me while I stroked his back and my clitoris at the same time. There was nothing for it. I needed more time but this wasn't the right place for it. He kissed my mouth, neck and cheeks and got up, rolled the condom off and pulled his trousers up while I scrabbled for my jeans and belt. I was trying to loop my belt back round my top, my jeans still lying on the floor, when Tall Boy slipped out to the bathroom to wash his hands and I heard his voice outside.

'Yes, of course,' I heard him say, 'I'll will print out those designs for you and have them with you in a minute.'

I froze. I didn't hear my boss's response but I didn't need to; my heart had stopped and I felt faint. What on earth was I doing in the spare office with the worst shag hair and no trousers? What would my boss say and had he heard us? We'd assumed the building was empty and hadn't exactly been quiet. Oh God, what if the other freelancer was back too?

I tried to be very, very quiet. Maybe I could sneak all the way downstairs and pretend I'd been out all the time. I peeked round the door and Tall Boy tried to signal to me, pointing to my boss's office. 'I'll bring those papers in a sec,' he said once more. 'Are you serious?' I mouthed, fumbling with my belt, my eyes wide with panic and the blood gushing in my head like the sound of a waterfall.

He nodded vigorously. I nearly cried. How effing stupid does one girl have to be? I *told* him I didn't conduct my affairs in the office! He might just be freelancing here, but I'm full time, this pays my mortgage and my taxes. And yet we'd gotten carried away.

Finally he started laughing. 'Arrrrrgh!' I screamed. 'You fucking bastard! I don't believe it!' and I ran at him, shunting him into the door frame and trying to slap his face in anger and relief.

He's thirty-two, not thirteen! Then he complained that I'd hurt his shoulder so I stopped pushing at him and we went for a post-coital lunch. In the street we bumped into my boss. 'Just grabbing a sandwich,' Tall Boy called and we sat on a bench with our food and laughed and teased each other. 'What did you do with the condom?' I asked him, and he pulled it out of his pocket, wrapped it in his empty sandwich box and tossed them in the bin.

Wednesday 6th June

For weeks I've been hoping that an ex-flatmate who lives close would help me take home the old TV that my boss wants to replace, but she recently confessed she's pregnant and feeling exhausted after work, so I didn't want to ask again. Of course, I didn't date KB just for his wheels, but he was always a great help when it came to things like this. I didn't expect Tall Boy to volunteer himself for the job.

'Are we getting rid of this thing, or what?' my boss asked with a sidelong glance at the TV. 'I still really want to take it home,' I replied as sweetly as I could, wondering if it would even fit in a taxi. 'I'll make sure I pick it up this week.'

'I've got a car,' Tall Boy piped up after the boss had gone to boil the kettle.

'Really? Will you drop if off for me?' I asked. I would never have thought that he possessed something as domestic as a car. With all his travel to far-away places I had assumed that anything without wings would be a really inconvenient method of transport.

'Would you really do that?' I asked him with a grin. 'Sure, I can come tomorrow after work.' 'Brilliant, thanks. You could take some of the old shelves you wanted for your house while we're at it.' Sorted.

Yesterday I stayed late – not realising that my boss would also still be around when Tall Boy turned up in his rickety car after office hours and sweated along with me to get the big monster into the boot. 'Oh, hi!' my boss called around the door, clearly surprised to see Tall Boy on a day when he wasn't working with us. 'He's come to pick up some of the old shelves,' I jumped in quickly before Tall Boy could tell him that I was the main reason for his drive across town on a Thursday night.

I nearly caught my finger as we pushed and pulled on the car seats; it really wasn't an easy task to fit in the TV together with the stand and the shelves. I held the boot door as he tied it all up with string, ready to go.

Lugging the telly across town and pushing it into place in my flat was sweet of him, but if he's interested in more than just a shag why can't we manage to go on something as uncomplicated as a date? At least he managed to stay for breakfast last time.

The signals are so mixed; maybe that ex of his really hurt him and he just needs time?

Friday 13th June

I had a belated barbecue birthday party at my flat this week. Tall Boy turned up with two friends and no card or present for me, just some free sweets he'd scored at another job and handed over. Imagine going to anyone's birthday, let alone someone you're sleeping with, and turning up empty-handed!

I should add that in the morning he'd been a real friend, driving me to the supermarket and helping me shop for party supplies. We got stuck in traffic and entertained ourselves singing along to the music while I stroked his neck. Still, I don't think it's too much to expect that he might have made time to write me a card before the party.

Anyway, one of his mates got off with one of my friends pretty early on, and Tall Boy and his American friend went off to another party. They returned at three-thirty a. m., and, woozy from booze and sleep, I opened the door to them and their two cans of beer. Then we all settled on the sofa with my new flatmate, who's only just moved here from Slovakia and was working hard on her English (we get on so well, she already feels more like a flatmate than a lodger).

The boys were meant to be massaging our feet, but Tall Boy was rubbish, making no effort whatsoever. After a while my flatmate retired, knackered by the effort of thinking in English and the breaking dawn outside. Tall Boy's friend trailed off in her wake. We heard her say, very plainly and flatly, 'I don't know you and I am going to bed alone. Good night.' And back he came. Wish I could put things so simply sometimes.

Not five minutes later, with the birds beginning to tweet, Tall Boy's friend picked up his mobile and dialled his fuck buddy. I sat there with my mouth hanging open at his brazenness. I could hear her chirpy replies to his probing questions as he wrangled to be invited over. 'Well, you'd regret it if I didn't see you tonight,' he said. Urgh.

I kicked him out. Tall Boy was snoozing on the sofa. I went to bed alone.

In the morning Tall Boy joined me in bed and stayed for breakfast, but somehow I felt almost as used as the other boy's fuck buddy.

Wednesday 20th June

Tall Boy was due back in the office this afternoon, so I texted him in the morning: 'It's hot and I fancy a swim – bring your trunks!' He turned up at lunch time with trunks but no towel, so we had to share mine.

After swimming a few lengths in the open-air pool, my goggled eyes steady on his wet form in the water, touching and kissing every time we reached the end of the pool, I climbed up the ladder and dried off. He was right behind me, cheekily cupping my bum, and we spread out my beach mat on the hot concrete and cuddled together, my head on his chest. I took my bikini top off to get a tan, aware I was giving the workers in the surrounding offices an eyeful.

'So, what are your plans for the summer?' I asked him as he stole glances at my nipples, and we reminisced about some of the countries we liked to visit. 'I'd like to take you with me to Portugal sometime, but not sure when . . . ' he trailed off. I wasn't sure if he was intentionally being vague, or just didn't want to turn up at his friend's wedding with me on his arm, which would surely prevent him from drinking his bodyweight in beer.

I could tell he was content just lying in the sun with me, stroking my arm before we had to get back to the office.

After work we went out with our respective mates and late in the evening I arranged to meet up with him. His friend had to rescue me from a hotel bar I'd wandered into in my confusion (his directions weren't great) and when I finally reached him, Tall Boy was really rather pissed. He hadn't come to fetch me himself because he was so pissed, in fact.

He kissed and cuddled me in front of his friends, bought me drinks and flirted, and we bantered about drinking, related minor criminal activities and odd places where we'd had sex. Then he got us a cab back to mine ('although you're welcome at my place, any time, you know that') because I had to be in the office early tomorrow. We frolicked on the sofa for a bit, and he was keen to get me into bed proper, so we retired and frolicked a bit more. And then he fell asleep and actually started snoring, still with his dick in my hand.

Which is pretty rude.

I sat astride him, his cock still hard on my palm, and briefly, idiotically, considered fucking him anyway, being horny, drunk and very annoyed, but then I realised that would be really damn weird.

I rolled over and tried to get some sleep, but couldn't. He pulled me towards him, spooning me and nuzzling my neck, but I wasn't in the mood for fake cuddles and pretend affection. So I did the 'logical' thing.

I picked up his blinking phone from the bedside table, and retreated to the bathroom like a cat with a half-dead canary.

And sure enough, curiosity killed the cat: there were messages explicit enough to confirm that:

+ He was sleeping with another woman at the end of May, long after our first shag.
+ It was her he went to see when he left my birthday party for a few hours, carrying a small goodbye gift as she was off to spend the rest of the year abroad.
+ They had got up to some naughty stuff in public a couple of weeks ago.
+ Some other girls seem to be quite fond of him too.
+ His sent box only stores five messages at a time so I gleaned most of my info from his messages received.

Yes, I felt bad. Maybe my insides dropped and my heart pumped a bit faster, but it didn't come as a massive surprise, just a confirmation of my instincts. Not like Pinocchio. There was no commitment, no fidelity or love or nonsense-shmonsense. My gut was right, although it was churning away now. Maybe I was a bit stupid and of course I resented the drunk, naked man sleeping in my bed, but what would he have found if he looked through *my* inbox?

Flirty texts from a raft of new dates, invitations to lunches and seduction attempts.

Yes, he wasn't honest, but then I never asked him anything that would have led him to lie. I found a photo of her on Bebo at work today, and she's like a complete physical opposite of me – height, skin colour, hair, shape, age. Her being so different from me has somehow made it easier to digest. And part of me is smiling – Tall Boy really is a match for me, we're as bad as each other! The difference is, I now really want to be in a committed relationship with the right person, and he doesn't, as he told me in the morning when we woke up and I asked him about the other girl. She's 'just a friend' he said, but I know better than that.

Despite all the booze I'd seen him consume the night before, he smelt like an angel and fucked like a god.

10

Doctors and Nurses

SUMMER 2007

Friday 29th June

I had to have a cone biopsy yesterday, owing to recurring abnormal cervical smears. The doctor showed me a tiny tissue sample they had snipped off my cervix – it bled a bit, but I am glad someone is taking care of it, even if I'm scared the big C might come and take my womb away before it's had the chance to fulfil its purpose. Ah, the privilege of being a medical volunteer. And hopefully future generations will get vaccinations against HPV and not have to go through this.

KB was back in touch. He lent me a friend's drill when I moved into my flat, and now he wants it back. No contact for three months, then you want your stuff back? Um, no mate. In other ex news, Pinocchio is getting married next week. And guess what? All I feel is relief that it's not me in the white veil.

Tall Boy phoned me at work to arrange when next to come into my office for business which 'does not concern my boss'. Unfortunately my boss was there to overhear our conversation, as were three other freelancers, so I'm sure we'll get found out sooner rather than later.

I need a holiday but I'm not sure whether to go on my own or with mates, or to take up one of my lovers on an offer.

Suggest I go to Portugal with Tall Boy? Fly to New York to see the Colonel and hope to escape with my anal virginity intact? I'd have to make him sign a contract to say he wouldn't attempt anything like that again. (After all I want to reserve *something* for my wedding night . . .)

Who says blondes with passports don't have fun?

Thursday 5th July

Now this is funny! Apparently Tall Boy rearranged his entire day so he could come to my office at lunchtime when there will be (a) no boss and (b) no freelancers hanging around. Except that, unbeknownst to him, there will also be (c) no Sienna. Because I seem to have missed the text he sent last night, and because I have a date with an Italian boy who's been hounding me on MSN.

I'm not going to let this Italian down just because Tall Boy's suddenly on the scene, so Tall will have to realise that I have other men in my life. Maybe he'll get jealous?

Monday 9th July

Last Thursday, Tall Boy came to the office to do his thing, and I just opened the door to him and rushed out to meet this Italian boy who's emailed me a picture of himself in his pants. As I dashed out I told him I hadn't got the text until too late, and the look on his face was priceless. Hah! Mind you, the lunch date was an utter washout.

I arrived five minutes late at the agreed location, and Mr Italian Underpants was nowhere to be seen. I called his phone. No answer. I wandered around some more, checking out the menus of various restaurants (they weren't exactly cheap –

hoped he was paying) and then decided just to sit down and have a coffee till he arrived.

Beep-beep went my phone. It was a text from him: 'I can see you.' Weird, I thought. Why doesn't he come up and say hello? Presumably he'll be with me in a second.

Beep-beep: 'Are you wearing red?' Well, yes. So he's got the right person. But where is he?

Beep-beep: 'Are you enjoying your coffee?' By now I was getting both annoyed and creeped out.

'Coward,' I texted back, a bit impatient because my stomach was growling and the mocha was vile.

Beep-beep: 'I don't think I am.' And yet, no sign of him.

I looked at my watch and saw it was half past one. I had wasted half an hour in an overpriced café in a draught, exchanging meaningless messages with a faceless freak. I called him again and this time he answered. 'Look,' I demanded, 'where are you? It's been thirty minutes and we wanted to meet for lunch. I'd like to eat now. What's going on? Why the strange messages?'

'Oh, ah, um,' he stammered, 'I'll be right there. Five minutes. Can you wait?'

I was incredulous, 'What do you mean, five minutes? You obviously saw me here, so why did you leave again?'

'Wait for me,' he pleaded, 'I'll be there.'

'No thanks,' I told him, 'this is stupid. I was here on time and you didn't even come up to meet me. I'm paying for my coffee and leaving. I can't be bothered with this. Bye.'

I made a quick getaway – not even a free lunch was worth being trapped with this freak. I found a cheaper café and cursed myself for not bringing a book. He called. I ignored it.

Beep-beep: 'Fine, so you are not going to wait for me, so you don't deserve me, but you are very beautiful, I'm sorry. Bye.'

Beep-beep: 'OK, you have all reasons to think I'm a monster.

I'm really sorry. You are beautyfull and you'll find a beautyfull man, sorry. Underpants Italian.'

Can you believe that this oddball manages to hold down a job in the City? On second thoughts, actually, I can believe that.

At least I had Tall Boy to go back to and sweeten my afternoon. We had a *delightful* day, in fact: after I'd entertained him with an account of my 'date', things got very interesting. I just can't keep my hands off this 'beautyfull' man (maybe Italian Underpants was right?) and just seeing his eyes across my desk made me happy.

Every time we went through some paperwork together he sneaked his arms round my waist, or I mussed up his hair or massaged his shoulders, although we made sure our work was done before we got down to business.

He pulled me towards him, onto my boss's chair, grasping me firmly as I slid my tongue into his mouth. He really is a wonderful kisser, although I'm a little haunted by the feeling that he's not 'all there' when our bodies merge and our hands meet. He seems mentally distracted and emotionally distant, which, given that fucking him and his beautiful, ever-hard cock could make me lose my job, is not so great. I've been here before (*sans* job concerns, but still).

I pushed the thought out of my mind as he yanked up my dress and fondled my breasts, then a new thought occurred – everyone in the office opposite could see what we were up to. 'We'll have a never-ending line of applicants for a job here tomorrow,' I joked as he laughed and pulled me to the floor.

We were grinding into each other, kissing hard and deep, his erect cock rubbing against my clit through our clothes. He got up to pull the blinds down and I pulled my leggings off. Then he stood over me, unbuckling his belt, as I knelt, ready for the release of his cock. I sucked him deeply, making him gasp. He turned me round and pulled my dress up again, on his knees, fondling my ass, my breasts, my pussy through my see-through black knickers and nudging the tip of his penis against my butt, trying to burrow between my ass cheeks.

'Are you on the Pill?' he asked and I had to admit that I wasn't. Out came the condom and I perched on my boss's desk while he rolled it on. He whipped my knickers off and I parted my legs, then he went down on me where I sat like a very naughty secretary indeed. When I couldn't stand it any longer and begged him to enter me, he fucked me as I lay back across the reports and the letters and the print-outs, utterly overwhelmed by the size of his cock and its sensation inside me.

Half sitting, I grasped his butt and pulled him into me, firmly, deeply and as hard as I could. I felt a slight discomfort – maybe the biopsy, or his size – and released my grip again, then he pulled out, bent me over the desk on my stomach and entered me roughly. The neighbours really would have got an eyeful, if it weren't for the blinds. Both naked now, we fucked like bunnies as the paperwork and paperclips scattered onto the floor and I crumpled up a spreadsheet in my hand, until he came with a huge groan, grasping me hard and kissing my back.

We collapsed on the floor and he held me as I stroked my clit, enjoying the afterglow. After a while we dressed, tidied up (I printed the spreadsheet out again) and raised the blinds. I had to go to a leaving do and he had to meet a friend, so we parted till Friday. Once again he said I'd be welcome at his house any time, but I think I'd rather have a specific invite or reason. After all, I'm not some kind of sexual pizza-delivery service.

Thursday 19th July

Why do I feel the need to confess in this blog? Am I confessing?

I've always written. It makes my life less confusing. And when

I was younger and finding out about sex for the first time, it was natural that I'd write about imagined sex too, with my friend Judy. We got gang-raped every weekend. How many teachers would suspect that a couple of twelve-year-old girls walking round the playground together eating their sandwiches would be talking about how their leather-clad biker boyfriends had lost them to the rest of the gang in a game of poker again? Or being ravished in their sleep by a man who'd been secretly in love with them for years?

This carried on till her mum found the letters, the books and the pictures of men in underpants we used to cut out of catalogues, and made Judy burn them. It was as if a world collapsed. She cried; I was deeply embarrassed. My mum never found out though – I think half those stories are still in her basement where I hid them. I must call Judy when I'm next home, and we can root them out and have a good laugh.

I have another little book now, as well as this blog. My tally is nudging forty. I wrote down their names, ages, nationalities and what we did, if it was love, an affair, a one-night stand. I think everyone has a little book like that somewhere.

Tall Boy is in the office today, working quietly. Too many people about. I'm chatting on MSN to a guy who enjoys being spanked and dominated. I have been the domme before, but I don't really enjoy it. Still, he's cute.

Friday 20th July

Tall Boy had some news for me last night.

My boss has found out about 'us'.

Not, I hope, by the strange marks on his desk or the crumpled paperwork, but for other reasons. After all, there's only so many times you can 'secretly' go swimming with someone in your lunch break, arrive at the office in their car because he was helping you 'pick up some furniture' or mention the things you do together after work before the penny drops in the thickest of skulls. And my boss isn't remotely thick.

So the other day, when I was off with a horrid stomach bug and Tall Boy asked my boss about me, he told Tall Boy:

'Sienna's off sick; why don't you call your girlfriend and ask her how she is?'

'Ahh, ha ha,' said Tall, not knowing what to say.

And then of course my boss caught me out having a drink with a friend that same evening, not being very sick at all anymore. That's probably a worse crime than dating Tall, but we're not an item after all and I don't want my boss to think I'm being unprofessional. At least we get our work done before anything happens.

If Tall Boy had told me about this little conversation sooner I wouldn't have pointedly reminded him about the play we were going to see last night within my boss's earshot. I bet he thought that was hilarious. Not that my evening with Tall Boy was anything special. I cooked him dinner, then we sweltered in the hottest theatre in London, flirted a bit and then he gave me a peck on the cheek and was off to meet a friend.

Not exactly romantic.

I think I need a change of scene. Found a last-minute deal for a yacht tour around the Greek Islands, maybe with some diving time. Hopefully the booking has gone through, then I'm out of here.

Monday 30th July

In the two years of writing this blog I have come to realise that it's not *less* disappointing to date four people who don't want to be emotionally involved, but *more* so. It's a numbers game: four unreliable guys are bound to piss you off four times as often as just one, even if you can always keep your options open with numbers five and six. I don't want to 'just have fun' any more or 'have sex like a man'. I want to have fun with the right person. Even if we can have mindless one-night stands, lusty fumbles, zipless fucks or drunken screws, secretly or not so secretly most women of childbearing age long for a man who will return our call the next day. Maybe mindless sex is just something for women to aspire to, but it grinds us down from the inside with each failed attempt. You wouldn't really go to bed with someone more than twice if there weren't something else that surpasses a mere physical attraction.

The situation with Tall Boy is causing me a lot of pain. He'd gathered that there wasn't going to be anyone but me in the office on Friday, so he was all keen to pop round and 'get some paperwork done' only I won't be there. Not another Italian Underpants date, but my holiday at long last.

I'm looking for a bit of space and blue sky to get Tall Boy out of my head. I have to break it off, it's getting toxic. Lust-sex feels fake now, with all those emotions bubbling under the surface and nowhere for them to go. I want to be in love and feel loved and have children as a happy by-product of that love.

Tall: Well, I thought we were having fun but if you're not happy with that then so be it.

Sienna: I try. I can't deny I'm having fun but it's not enough for you and not enough for me.

Tall: Well, I had a girlfriend for two years and now I want to be single.

Sienna: Man logic! But I understand. Men want to have their cake and eat it, and us girls are dumb enough to

serve it to them. Mind you, I don't want to be a girlfriend.

Tall: Just a wife, eh?

Sienna: Or lovers. Girlfriend/boyfriend is so schizo. Good
that you're not jealous, otherwise that would really
complicate things! [I couldn't resist that little dig.]

Tall: Indeed. Did I mention that I'm someone who loves
shagging you?

I can't win. He's handsome, charming, horny, unreliable and
happily single. And I want to fuck his brains out. Thank God
I'm going to be out of the office, and the country.

Wednesday 15th August

Back from my yacht trip around Greece and feeling – how shall
I put this? – healed? By a pair of magical doctors and two weeks
of sea salt in the air and sand under my feet. Maybe I can fuck
like a man after all, or at least I can when I'm on holiday from
my life, my flat, my office, my boss and my Tall graphic
designer. And they really were both doctors – surgeons, in fact,
but I'm getting ahead of myself here.

Doctor number one was actually the mate of a guy I really
fancied, a gorgeous, tall Dutchman. That one had a girlfriend of
four years, but he invited me along to spend the evening with his
crew the night we reached another, even more beautiful island. I
went alone, as the rest of my group wanted an early night.

I joined his gang and we sat and had cocktails in an amazing
cliff-top bar. As we all chatted away, I found myself intrigued by
two of his friends, one of them a guy who worked in music
publishing, the other a surgeon from Amsterdam who used to
want to be a fireman. After an hour or so, the boys wanted to

move on to a cheesy club but I had other plans. I'm a club aficionado in London, and if I can go to the best nightspots at home, why do I want to go somewhere crap on a tiny island when I can sit out all night and watch shooting stars over a clear, peaceful sea?

I told them I'd walk out along the cliffs instead. They bid me goodnight and trotted off, but Dr X held back. 'Would you like some company?' he offered. It was too dark to check if he was really my type or not (I suspected not) but I appreciated his sweet offer and he followed me down the cliff path to the platform where I'd swum and snorkelled earlier with my boat mates.

I don't remember who suggested swimming – not me, I think, as I'd just painstakingly washed my hair in the cramped and sweltering on-board bathroom – but, happy and drunk on shooting stars and ice-blended cocktails, I whipped my dress off over my head and jumped into the dark water head first.

'Is it safe?' Dr X asked from above. 'I have operated on a lot of people who broke their necks diving into shallow water.'

'Of course it is, silly,' I shouted up to him, 'I was here earlier and you can see the bottom in daylight. It's six metres deep.'

And he jumped in after me feet first.

We swam round the base of the cliffs and into a cave where our movement through the water lit up millions of tiny phosphorescent algae, giving our limbs a sparkly green submarine glow. It was magical. Out of the cave, I floated on my back and saw another five shooting stars, running out of wishes as I watched them zoom across the sky in quick succession.

Dr X floated near me and we locked together like two floating starfish, his feet near my armpits and mine on either side of his shoulders, and we held onto each other, staring up. It was the loveliest, cosiest position. I could have fallen asleep like that. His body cupped mine in the water, warming me and making me feel safe and happy, and he began stroking my feet. I didn't reciprocate much, as I didn't know where this would lead, but I just revelled in it and the sky above.

A million, billion stars in a sky blacker than you'd ever see it in light-polluted London . . . I felt a bit cold after a while and climbed back up the cliff onto a ledge, my white undies shining in the darkness. Dr X followed close behind and hugged me to him, nuzzling my neck. Then he turned me round and kissed me, salt water dripping off our faces and bodies, lapping and probing at my mouth.

I didn't particularly like his kissing but its urgency made me horny and I tried to catch at his lips and steer his tongue till he was getting it right. His hands were roaming my body, and he unhooked my bra and dipped his head to suck my nipples. I could feel his erection against my leg, hot behind his cold, wet underpants, and one of his hands slipping down to my pants. I gasped in anticipation and felt his fingers push between my lips and his intake of breath when he felt the warmth of my pussy against the cold, wet material of my knickers. He stripped them off me and I kicked them away, followed by my bra and his pants.

I was beginning to get dry and the wind was chilly, and I was suddenly aware that the teenage Greek kids I'd seen earlier in the evening might look down on us, so I pulled my dress on again. Dr X pushed me against the rock face, grasping my waist from behind, and I braced myself with one hand while the other rubbed my clit. He reached under me to push himself into me, but I stopped him. Wouldn't you think a doctor knew better than to fuck strange women on cliffs without protection? I grabbed a condom from my handbag and held the silver packet up. 'What luck!' I pretended, rather than dare admit that I'd come prepared on purpose.

I faced the rocks again and braced myself, and he pushed my dress up and thrust his cock into me, which felt so good that I broke into a smile, then panted and pushed against him as he fucked all the tension and frustrations out of me.

Somehow the condom came off but I provided a second one, and he laid me back on the ground before lowering himself over me. We tried a few different positions on the stairs and the rocks but gave up anything other than standing up, after my back and his knees got grazed. I came and he did soon afterwards – over quickly but it was just too horny.

We lay back on the stairs leading up to the path and laughed about how naughty we'd been. Soon he began stroking me again, his hand roaming . . . His neck tasted salty. When I felt how hard he was again I was turned on all over again, and took his glistening cock in my mouth which he enjoyed enormously, judging by his comments and the noises he made when he couldn't do words any more.

He went down on me, mumbling appreciation of how shaved and soft I was, then he was inside me again, me crouched over him, riding him . . .

We walked back to my boat together and parted, me to sleep, him to join his mates. He kissed me to try and placate me, but didn't ask for my number. I told him to get it from his friend. Oh well, it was a bit of an anticlimax, but it did leave a smile on my face. And now, typing about it, I have to go and have a quick play with myself before I explode!

Tuesday 21st August

On my last night, a French Doctor who lives in Athens, who'd been advising me about my trip before I left London via a social networking site, took me for cocktails and then dinner on the roof terrace of a hotel. We watched the remains of the sunset playing over the Acropolis, and looked out all the way to the sea. I ordered a lobster risotto and a glass of Rossini and the conversation flowed, and by the time we were spooning up our sorbet the flirtation was heating up.

At first, I didn't fancy him in the least as he's not what I'd call my usual type – shortish, somewhat skinny, thinning hair and dark eyes, he smokes – and yet he was also genuine, nice, normal and generous. If you could ignore the Marlboro, he smelt of nice aftershave and he paid me plenty of compliments in a sexy French accent with an honest, sweet smile. He was seriously interesting to talk to as well and listened intently before giving good advice.

He specialised in breast surgery. It was interesting to get his opinion on the big C (my aunt died of breast cancer) and vain girls and transsexuals who get their boob jobs on the NHS. Later he drove me back to my hotel in the Plaka, and I made him put the top down on his convertible. I arrived at the door with mad hair and a big smile, tired but a little disappointed at having to go to bed at a reasonable time. I bade him goodnight and decided to wander round the shops that were still open.

My phoned beeped and it was a text from the French Doctor: 'If you are not tired, would you like to join me at my place for a night swim?' I struggled with myself a bit. After all, I had an early flight to catch and was plunging straight back into work in London. On the other hand, I wasn't *that* tired, and even though it was getting dark it was 34 degrees. One last swim would be perfect. Plus I wanted to see the inside of his house. Pure curiosity.

I texted a 'yes please' and bought some frappé lattes for us to sip on the drive to the suburbs of the city, and he swooped up in the car and off we went.

The convertible wound its way into a leafy street and up to a set of gates which opened automatically. Inside we parked the car and got out to a welcome from a knot of cute little kittens and a dog barking greetings. He loves animals. Home!

In the garden he cracked open a bottle of Baron Rothschild Chardonnay and poured us each a glass before disappearing to try and find his trunks while I chased the dog round the pool. No luck locating the Speedos, so as I slid into the pool in a sparkly bikini he stripped down to his underpants and climbed in. And the underpants immediately became see-through. I tried not to look, obviously, but his body looked a lot more appealing without the clothes. Not skinny as much as really fit and toned, with firm abs and biceps.

Relaxing in the cool water with this attentive, tanned man while his cute dog ran around the edge, I asked him what the most bizarre thing was he'd ever seen in the hospital. 'Well,' he began, 'a man in a pin-striped suit. A very respectable, business type of guy in his forties. He told me he wasn't gay, but that two of his girlfriends had come round the other night with some coke, and left a huge double-ended dildo in his arse!'

I couldn't believe it and burst out laughing, I mean, I'd always assumed these stories were urban legends, but he assured me they were all true. He held his hands a foot apart to show me how long it had been. 'The nurses were taking photos! We get this all the time. Fish, a showerhead, a cucumber, all sorts!'

And I thought women were inventive! He paddled closer and pulled me into one of the nicest kisses I'd ever experienced. Even the taste of tobacco didn't turn me off – for once it reminded me of Pinocchio in a good way, making my body think of all the fun sex we used to have. I felt a bubble of lust welling up. Bad idea, I thought, remember your early flight, think how you'll feel if he never gets in touch again, and stick to your new principles: if you are beginning to like someone, wait until you know he loves you before you sleep with him. Look after your heart.

We'd had a fun evening with great conversation, and I was hoping this could turn into more if we got to know each other properly. The Dutch doctor had been different, all I'd been interested in him for was his ability to make me come, but with the French Doctor I saw the potential for more than just a one-night stand. I pushed him away with a smile and we both climbed out of the pool, only when I saw him standing there like a Greek statue wrapped in just his towel, and remembered his delicious dick against my thigh in the water, I just had to have him. Why the heck not? Thoughts crept into my head as I got slowly turned on by the possibilities in store: 'I'm in a hot country drinking delicious wine with a delectable doctor, I'm free and single, this is impossibly romantic, it's the end of my holiday, I might regret it if I backed away now when I'm old and wrinkly in a rocking chair.'

'I can drop you back any time,' he reassured me. 'Just say the word.'

'I will, but not quite yet.' I'd only meant to stay till midnight and now it was past that. Once again, my libido overruled my reason. Will I ever be able to stick to my own rules?

We talked about relationships, the difference between male and female attitudes and about love. 'If you are older than sixteen you can't fall in love properly,' I told him. 'You need a certain degree of naivety for that, and you're too cynical once you're past that age.'

'Why?' he asked. 'Can't we always fall in love as if we're teenagers?'

A lovely thought, I agree, but unrealistic. Or is it? From his lips, uttered with conviction and warmth, it didn't sound like 'just a phrase'. 'There's an island with a church where we can get married,' he teased, cueing visions of me in white silk with a gaggle of tanned, happy kids who learn to swim in sea water as clear as glass.

'Yeah right,' I said, but I pulled him down and gave him a wet kiss on the lips.

He held a towel open for me and I climbed out of the pool to let him dry me as the dog jumped round us, excitedly.

I took my glass of wine indoors and sat down in the living room, and the Doctor followed me in and sat astride my lap. Not the most erotic thing for a man to do, I admit, but it made me laugh and was strangely sexy when he started kissing me. 'A lap-dancing doctor? I like that.' I kissed him back.

His lips wandered down to my chest and his finger began teasing my nipple through the wet bikini top. 'Don't you get enough tits at the office?' I asked him. 'I like to see you get excited,' he replied, hoarsely, and started to pull my top down.

Talk about performance anxiety – I waited till I was twenty-five for the boobs I thought I'd grow, with no results. My boobs aren't exactly small and they're perky and firm, but compared to the rest of me (i.e. my butt) they are disappointingly small. And now they were being contemplated by a breast specialist.

His tongue found my nipple and he stroked and caressed me as I wondered exactly how far we were going to go, but when his hand unknotted my towel and plunged into my bikini bottoms I felt my pussy respond with enthusiasm. He lured me to a bed in an alcove and spirited my bikini top right off – an expert in bra clasps too. His towel had been left trailing on the floor and I could feel his hard-on, a warm hunk of excited flesh, against my leg.

His penis pushed against my bikini bottoms, stretching them into my pussy. He leapt up to get some condoms, then pulled my bikini down, teased my legs apart and lowered his head into my lap. As he licked at me he turned on the bed so his knees were by my ears. I hadn't done sixty-nine for a long time – there are few things less attractive than a perineum in close-up – but his impressive cock was just begging to be sucked. I licked at it as his tongue pounded my clit with a steady rhythm, then I slid his long, thick cock as far as I could down my throat. Funny, he was skinny enough to sit on my lap, but with this surprise in his pants.

He turned again on the bed and slid himself slowly into me, right to the end, making me gasp as I was still a little sore from Doctor X on the cliffs, but I was so wet and horny that after a few thrusts I opened up and pulled him fully into me, grasping his buttocks and sucking his neck as he kissed my breasts. 'Play with yourself,' he insisted, although I didn't need any encouragement. I came quickly and then he came straight away, then I came again, shivering and clenched round him as he pumped the condom full of warm sperm.

He rolled off and reached for me, placing my head on his chest and lazily stroking my back. My hand rested on his flat, tanned stomach and we caught our breath. 'I could fuck you all night,' I told him. 'Why don't you then?' he challenged me.

Suddenly we heard the noise of chatting and laughing outside. It was his neighbours, who must have heard everything through the open French windows.

'That's embarrassing,' I said.

'I don't care,' he laughed and I looked up to see him grinning. He got up to remove the condom and fetch his cigarettes, then smoked two, leisurely, his legs resting on mine. If someone lights up next to me on a park bench I usually move away, but for some reason this was OK.

We began playing again, and this time I went on all fours, gagging for him, a little sore but desperate to be fucked hard.

'Baby' he called me as he pulled my hair and pounded away, with my hands playing on my clit and his balls. He sneaked a thumb cheekily into my butt hole, nearly pushing me over the edge, but I held back to enjoy the sensation of him ramming into me, and then he came. I missed my orgasm but was so close that I groaned loud enough to end the neighbours' conversation. We collapsed back onto the sheets, breathless and laughing about the neighbours, and his dog going ape-shit outside the door. Then the conversation turned from jokes to Greek drama and philosophy as we drowsed, his cigarette smoke curling up and out of the French doors, our bodies naked under the sheets. I ruined it all by glancing at my watch: 'It's four ! Shit!'

He dropped me off at my hotel with a lingering kiss and an invitation to Santorini, and I turned in for three hours' sleep and some frantic packing.

Let's hope September yields some cheap flights!

11

New Babies, Old Feelings

AUTUMN 2007

Tuesday 28th August

The night before we got back to Athens I had a text from Samantha, my ex-best friend. It read: 'I heard you got a lovely new flat, I also have big news. I moved house and had a baby!'

At the time it felt like a punch in the gut. The holiday was nearly over, I'd only gotten one scuba dive in and I was surrounded by people who were mates but not friends. I don't know why it unsettled me so much – I don't wish her ill but I was genuinely shocked, surprised and also, I realised, pleased for her. I went to the beach on my own then sobbed, feeling like an unholy mess with conflicting emotions. Then I texted back: 'Congratulations. I can't believe it! Who's the daddy?'

It turned out that it was a guy she'd met through a dating site and had only known for three weeks when she fell pregnant. They weren't together any more. She sent a photo, but I couldn't open it while I was abroad so our conversation stopped for a week or so.

I wanted to go and see the new one – I'm a sucker for babies and they flock to me like the proverbial flies – but I had a few reservations. She used to get me to look after her cat for free when she was on holiday then complain that I hadn't hoovered up all the cat hair, as though I was meant to be her maid. Does she just want a cheap babysitter? Or is she bored with her new life? Have her party-loving friends turned their backs now she's a single mum?

I trotted off to see them on Saturday, ready to have my heart softened. I took flowers and a humungous teddy that my Sweet Ex got me, which is utterly wasted on me.

It was odd having her open the door to her new flat with the little one in her arm. It was odd that she didn't know how to hold his head. Strange how quickly it all happened for her and the father, a penniless giant who lives in a flat share in Cambridge. What a shame she went off him as soon as she got pregnant and told him to leave just after he got her the cheapest ring Tiffany would yield (*sans* diamond). Odd how she expected to live off the £60 a week he can afford to give them.

She had moved in two weeks before, and the flat was still a mess with the baby crib in pieces and the nursery unpainted. I sat down and held him while she made us coffee. Two years' worth of the biggest changes in our lives were told in under thirty minutes: my flat, KB, my new job, her ex, her new flat, her pre-eclampsia and emergency caesarean, rushed through in a flurry of rediscovery.

The baby smiled up at me and I stroked his soft skin and hair. He was quite happy, even though he'd only just met me and I'd interrupted his lunch. She took him back and resumed nursing, telling me she'd only realised the lounge had no direct sunlight after she moved in . . .

I suggested a walk to the park as it was sunny for the first time since he was born, and she was happy to get out of the flat. I pushed the pram on the way to the park, feeling like a proud new mum. On our way back she pushed it and I got cat-called by a bunch of builders in a van. Funny how getting covered in your friend's regurgitated breast milk can begin to heal old wounds.

Thursday 30th August

Multi-dating never works how you'd like it to. Either the men crowd you all at once or they just disappear off the face of the earth simultaneously.

French Doctor has been suspiciously quiet. No more talk of Santorini but he confirmed there were nasty fires in Athens; it seemed to worry him, not surprisingly. According to his online profile, Porsche Boy is 'in a relationship' with a Latvian beauty born in – wait for it – 1985. What a cradle-snatcher! Canada Boy found some pictures of us in London and posted them on his site – how lovely, and what great memories. I came over all sentimental. I miss that boy. We still have long MSN conversations.

Yacht Boy resurfaced and invited me for a weekend's sailing as he's 'less busy at work' – he has turned twenty-nine and bought a new boat. I wondered where he'd been in the meantime. I might as well go, but I'm worried because I've met this boy exactly twice in my life. What is he thinking? Apparently his brother and *his* girlfriend are coming too, although in their own boat. I don't feel threatened by the prospect of staying the night with him, just a bit daunted as I don't know him well.

Tuesday 4th September

The weekend started a little earlier than I'd anticipated. I was planning an early night on Friday in preparation for an early start with my trip with Yacht Boy, so instead of pissing about in the West End I invited a select group of friends over to mine for an impromptu barbecue to make the most of one of the last nice evenings of the year.

One of the people I invited was my flatmate's friend, Fencing Boy. He had been a very patient suitor of hers, who'd been rejected by her at every turn in that friendly, inoffensive way of hers. She just doesn't fancy him enough, or some such nonsense.

After I met him for the first time I tried to persuade her otherwise. He is perfectly charming, good-looking, posh and intelligent with a hint of arrogance about him. He cuts a nice figure in a suit and the chat was all about his love of travelling and the business he was building. He told me he was sure I'd been to a finishing school, which I let him believe for about five minutes, telling him it was in Switzerland, hence my faint accent. Then I came clean and told him I didn't even know what they taught in finishing schools. 'How to walk with good posture and get out of a car without flashing your knickers,' he told me confidently. 'You don't need a teacher to do that,' I said, 'you just keep your legs together.'

I found him sweet though, and asked my flatmate how she could turn him down, but she wasn't coming round. 'If you like him so much, *you* have him,' she said, and I said that was silly and that those sorts of things – recycling boyfriends – never worked out. 'No, go for it,' she prodded me, and gave me his number.

So that explains his presence at the barbecue and our nice chat over a good rosé. When my guests started to feel cold I led them all in to the sofa and the telly, and we chatted and drank merrily and it stopped being an early night and turned into a civilised sort of party. Eventually everyone had gone and my flatmate had retired to bed, leaving only Fencing Boy wrestling with a faulty DVD on the sofa.

Then he pounced. It was a full-on, horny snog, taking me by surprise, but very, very welcome. I worried about the open living room door, but no one came in and his kisses grew more urgent. I loved every second of it and didn't stop his hands as they smoothed my cheeks and then slid up my skirt. I guess I was pretty drunk but here was a boy who'd risked outright rejection by planting the first kiss and whom I knew I fancied, and who turned out to be a fantastic kisser.

I was getting wet and knew we wouldn't have our clothes on for much longer. I got up to shut the door then returned to the sofa and sat astride him. He unhooked my bra and pulled my top off, then fell on my nipples, kissing and sucking them. I sighed and he pushed me over on my back, grinding against me as I clutched at and scratched his back.

My fingers reached for his belt and he pushed my skirt up and whipped my knickers off in one fast movement, then dived between my thighs. He licked and sucked till I was on the point of coming, slipping his finger in and out of my wetness, his tongue tickling my clit as I tried to stop myself from crying out (thank goodness a CD was playing).

His head bobbed up and he looked at me. I reached for his belt again. 'Do you want to?' he asked as his cock sprang free. I could feel the smooth, warm hardness of it against my wet thighs, and I didn't care if he fucked me right then and there, just like that. He lifted himself off me to reach for his wallet and a condom and I took the opportunity to assess his cock and take it in my mouth. He whimpered, 'Ooh that feels so great,' and I went on sucking him deeply till I think he was getting worried he would come in my mouth. Then I pulled back so he could roll the condom on. Then he was over me again, holding my hand in his and kissing me, his cock entering me slowly.

I pulled him in so he fucked me faster, right there on the sofa with his jeans round his ankles. We were both topless and writhing together, slick with each other's saliva. The look on his face was pure tenderness and passion and we came at nearly the same time.

He held my face in his hands and told me he thought I 'rocked' but it really touched me. 'Oh, such beautiful breasts,' he said, examining them closely for the first time. 'I didn't see them properly before.'

I hadn't even stopped to think whether it would be a good idea to sleep with him, and what this might imply, I simply let myself get swept up. Plus it always feels so good when someone I fancy actually fancies me back and pounces. Being seduced is one of my all-time fantasies, and, like a box of chocolates, once that lid is off there's no stopping me. It's not as if I had planned this and expected anything, so who knows where this might lead – the orgasm and the unselfconscious way we'd both let ourselves go reminded me that as long as my heart's not tied up elsewhere I can still enjoy as much guilt-free sex as I want.

We giggled together as we surveyed the damage done by the glass of whisky and Coke we'd upended in the throes of passion and he let me kiss his shoulders as he wrapped the condom up in tissue. He had tiny white acne scars on his back that looked like water drops and I kissed them and told him I thought they were cute.

'Not when you're a teenager,' he remarked.

'No teenager ever feels cute,' I replied.

Wednesday 5th September

Just in case you didn't know, sailing is very sexy. The movement of the boat is almost like a living thing, a large sea horse, a strong man, an overpowering wave. Which accounts for me being a little bit frustrated after my weekend with Yacht Boy.

I woke up on Saturday morning a little surprised to be so

chipper and excited about meeting Yacht Boy after my tipsy night with Fencing Boy. I had to wear a silk scarf around my neck to hide the huge love bite he had left behind. When I got off my train and met Yacht Boy at the station he was bright-eyed and bushy-tailed too, and I sat in the car while he got us some coffees. We had plenty to talk about and I tried not to let my annoyance at having heard nothing from him for so long creep into the conversation. All was hunky-dory, fluffy and fun. It set the tone for the weekend.

We got to the boat and found his brother and girlfriend, then lugged the provisions on board and set off down the estuary. Within ten minutes of lifting the anchor I was steering – he obviously trusted me with control of his prized possession.

A pleasant two days followed. On the Saturday we went to a gig on the Isle of Wight, then cuddled up in the 'master cabin'. He pulled my head onto his chest, but even though we'd got a bit touchy-feely and very flirty during the day and evening, nothing happened apart from a few snogs. The poor boy was tired and I didn't want him to think I was easy, or a raging nymphomaniac for that matter.

The rocking of the boat and the wine made me quite horny though, and I lay there moistening and listening to his sleepy breathing and rapidly getting frustrated. I wondered about the possibility of a lazy morning shag. It was so intimate to be lying there together squashed into the berth but there was a huge distance between us. I couldn't forgive him quite so easily for the long silence between Easter and now. At six, when the sun and the seagulls woke us up, I tried to rouse his interest by stroking his hand in a subtle, seductive way, but he just went back to sleep. His brother woke us at 10 and we were required on deck so that was that.

Sailing back to the mainland was a bit of an adventure: the

sea and wind picked up and I found myself helming the boat at eight knots, battling strong winds and a choppy sea. Still, I managed to make us a late brunch breakfast when Yacht Boy took over, serving up scrambled eggs, bacon and toast. Luckily I'd developed my sea legs in Greece. We got back to port under a gloomy late-afternoon sky and I stripped down to my bikini and jumped into the chilly water for a refreshing dip. 'I can't believe you actually went in,' said Yacht Boy, rushing to the side as he heard the splash, and as I climbed back up the ladder, 'Gosh, you look just like that Bond Girl.'

Back at his parents' house I had a shower but he ignored my subtle hints to join me, then we had a slap-up dinner. On our way back to London we laughed and joked, keeping him awake when he was worn out with fresh sea air. He dropped me at the train station with a smile and a kiss. And an invitation for a further trip this month.

I must remember that I am trying to find a guy I actually want to be with, and not waste time making it too easy for guys who just want a brief fling, so although I was horny on the boat I don't regret not sleeping with him yet. I'll wait and see if he actually calls me about that next trip. What I was thinking when I let myself be seduced by Fencing Boy, I just don't know – maybe old habits dic hard – but I like him too and it was fun . . .

I think the difference between my two encounters this weekend is that one was totally spontaneous, unplanned, a spur-of-the-moment thing without the pause for thought. Now, of course, I wonder what is going to happen with Fencing Boy, if he sees any potential for 'us', or whether, indeed, I do. I don't think I know enough about him yet. All I know is that fucking him felt great and didn't leave me too confused and vulnerable. If nothing further comes out of it, it was just that – a fun fuck between friends.

Yacht Boy, however, is a different matter. When we first met he seemed keen and interested in a relationship, but then his calls just dried up. I think a little bit of effort and consistency is required if there is some kind of plan involved, so I am understandably wary. Not sleeping with him too soon is the only way to protect my heart when all these expectations have been building up based on the way he acted when we first met. Of course if nothing actually happens I am left wondering if he just doesn't fancy me enough? After all there's a difference between pushing away someone who is trying to take things too fast (there's always a chance to yield to his advances if I felt like it) and wondering whether someone fancies me any more if he doesn't try it on at all. Or perhaps he was just showing respect?

All I know is that I have got to try and go the path of the least emotional hurt whilst still enjoying my single status with all its advantages like horny, uncomplicated sex and weekend sailing tips.

Confused? So am I!

Thursday 6th September

Maybe I shouldn't have gone to the cinema with Tall Boy last night. Or to the park at lunch time. Maybe I need to wear body armour that will give him an electric shock every time he touches me. Maybe I need to go on methadone or some other type of replacement drug. Maybe I should never touch his hair again, or shrink from his kisses.

Maybe I should tell him I'm in love with him.

Then what?

To everyone around us in public we must look like the perfect couple. Tall, striking, smiling, tactile. Me buying the cinema tickets, him springing for the popcorn and drinks, sharing the bag, the straw, laughing.

Maybe it's this lightness he likes, the lack of expectations. I try to remember not to question him, keep it breezy, be his mate, his lover; the woman whose hand he holds in the dark. Those lips, so firm and strong, the soft, probing tongue, perfect suction. I never had a problem kissing him, not the way you have to teach some men how to kiss – not slobbering, spinning your tongue around like a broken washing machine or trying to eat you, just kiss; give, take, smile, break, kiss again more softly, passion growing, biting lips, not a set pattern you learned from your ex.

We sit and he strokes my hair, and this stolen moment is so precious although the film really sucks. A boys' film, and I can't help but laugh out loud at it, but mainly I'm smiling because I'm happy he is here with me.

He likes to be spontaneous, and I snatch these moments when I can, and it doesn't feel forced. I wish I was able to hold back better, let him come chase for a change. We seem to fall into these intimate patterns quite naturally – like sitting in the park with our sandwiches, my bare legs crossed under my skirt, him stretched out on the lawn. Too close to be 'just friends'. I can smell him, and he is wearing a smart shirt with those beaten-up old jeans I remember unbuttoning. He sniffs my neck and tells me he loves my scent. I curl my fingers into his soft hair and he sighs with pleasure.

We don't talk about anything of significance. Friends, shopping, travelling, languages, that sort of thing. His house, my flat. Work. My mad boss and his silent partner, who gets so frustrated with him he doesn't stay silent when he calls me on the phone to complain.

Tall Boy freelances at other companies and tells me about the crazy creative types he comes into contact with, or the dull and dowdy ones who need his services but wouldn't know creativity if it came and sat in their hair.

I've finished my lunch and curl up next to him, both looking up into the sky with my head resting on his bicep.

I try to tie myself to these moments, since I cannot tie these moments to me.

Tuesday 11th September

Under topaz London skies I dive into my oasis of blue, surrounded by hunky men in trunks and the odd patch of sunlight. The water calms me and the close-ups of strangers' cellulite reassures me in an odd way.

I bake on the terraces, watching the men, wishing for a strong boy's body, bronzed, about nineteen years old I'd say, so I could cruise them properly. Or a tall and slightly paunchy body with wide shoulders and chest hair, like my Tall Boy's.

Tall Boy has reported back from the locker rooms, telling me what's going on between the men there. I'm curious to know if the same thing happens in a semi-public place in London between men and women too. He's mentioned that he's intrigued by a well-known sauna which is essentially a swingers' club. Will I go with him? I think I'd be too jealous. Who wants to see their ideal guy (well, he would be if it wasn't for that thing between his ears) cosying up to some size-ten beauty? Or old ladies lusting after his perfect dick? Who wants to watch him watching me get fucked by someone whose face I don't care to see again?

As I basked in the sunshine after work in my bikini yesterday, something odd happened: My eye snagged on a man's crotch close by. He was grabbing it. First, it looked like he was just resting his hand on his crown jewels. I thought: 'What an apish, nasty macho pose, does he think he's alone in his bedroom?' and tried to concentrate on my book.

Then it became more obvious what he was doing, or maybe trying not to do.

There were two Turkish girls in their late teens next to me, and this hairy, chubby guy with the crotch-grabbing obsession kept checking them out, then looking down at his crotch, before 'subtly' re-adjusting himself. It became harder to take my eyes off it, as he became harder (or was it just my imagination?) He gave it one more tug, then got up and stared at the swimming pool, then sat back down again and checked out his willy's private life.

He went so far as to lift his waistband, and look at it. I was disgusted, and considered getting up to complain. 'There is a man touching himself over there,' I would say to the lifeguard, and watch as he was escorted from the premises.

Instead, I kept watching him. Was what he was doing truly indecent? Was it intentionally exhibitionist, or just casually careless? And – I got turned on. The outline of his stiffening cock in the sun, his occasional stroking or grabbing of it, and his sweaty, swarthy body began to send tingles into my moistening pussy.

I could make out its size and the head, and the balls below quite clearly, and it seemed to be growing.

I don't know why I had such a strong physical response. Intellectually, I was disgusted and should have been outraged, but instead I found myself wishing for an alternative universe where I could beckon him over with a flick of my eyelashes and a flash of a nipple, and have him come over to me, hot from the sun, pushing me onto my knees, pull down my bikini, and enter me swiftly, followed by hard, merciless strokes as people around us watched him give me a good seeing-to.

He'd come with a groan (I'd be glad I wouldn't be able to see his face), drip the last drops of his cum onto my bare buttocks as he pulls out of me, give his dick a quick squeeze and tug it back into his shorts. Without a backward glance, he'd return to his sun-drenched corner, whilst I'd lie back and then go for a refreshing swim. Like monkeys in the zoo.

Is this ever going to happen? Would people really do this? *Did* they do it, back in prehistoric times? Why did the outline of a stranger's cock give me the female equivalent of a stiffy, apropos of nothing?

If I had spoken even one word to him, my whole turned-on-ness would have collapsed like a house of cards. He was SO NOT my type. It was just his cheeky, bold, fucking dick that did it. Fuck, I am turned on now I am typing this.

I am irritatingly sexually charged at the moment, to the point that I have one-night stands in my dreams: the sex is graphic, sweaty and random, and I wake up desperate for a morning boner in bed next to me. Fat chance. If I can have no-strings-attached lusty sex in my fantasies, why can't I do it in real life?

I'm back to what I had before: an assortment of men, each perfect and flawed in their own way and none of them willing to commit. When I started multi-dating, having all this atten-tion and sex lavished on me seemed like the perfect cure for Pinocchio, but when I look back at my old blog entries all that talk about 'having sex like a man' seems incomprehensible. Did I really believe that? Instead I'm discovering that with each encounter at least one of my heartstrings stays firmly attached to the guy: BBP, the Pilot, Cashmere, Kensington . . . Giving in to my libido unfortunately doesn't prevent me from getting hurt: instead I am finding that all the great orgasms don't make up for the disappointment I feel when I'm let down again, and that all the caresses that stroke my ego sadly leave my heart neglected. I wish I could find someone able to satisfy both my pussy and my heart.

And work is going into uproar again. My boss has decided to move the company to the outskirts of London and I don't fancy the commute, so I had better hit 'situations vacant' again.

Monday 24th September

I don't understand why some employers appear not to want someone intelligent, interesting, articulate and educated to man their offices, instead of someone quiet, boring and slightly dumb with minimum typing skills. I'm getting turned down for jobs because I 'may not find it stimulating enough'. My current job is hardly stimulating most of the time (unless Tall Boy is in the office!)

Why do recruitment companies call and ask you what you are looking for, only to trip you up when you say you're building a career in one industry and offer you a job in another industry? And how does anyone keep a straight face when being interviewed by a twenty-eight-year-old MD who tries to rattle you with 'business speak' only to be unable to translate it when you politely ask him to elaborate?

Love-life news? Well, there's not much. Fencing Boy and I had an explosive night together after a gig in Soho and I lured him into the shower as a prelude to a good roll in my bed. After a little misunderstanding when I asked him what his little finger was doing inside me and he took it as an invitation to insert it into my anus, I found myself being explored for certain other 'back passage pleasures'. What is it with posh boys and rimming? I wonder if he thinks I'll return the favour. In any case, it was very nice and as we fucked I felt that we were equally passionate, giving people who moved in unison, bathed in each other's sweat. Oh, and we broke the bed. The new bed.

I love talking to him as much as I love fucking him and we chatted as we waited for his taxi. He asked me if I used to be into riding. 'Um, no,' I said. 'Only recently, and the horse can usually tell I have no experience and bolts with me.' My parents had never been able to afford for me to have riding lessons, so the only ponies I got to sit on were rocking horses, hobby horses and nags at the fairground.

'So you didn't win that,' he pointed at a pink rosette pinned by the bed.

'Not really,' I took it off the curtain for closer inspection. It read: BIRTHDAY GIRL.

So much for that. I think he must have been labouring under the delusion that I'm posh too, with my imaginary finishing school and my imaginary pony.

Wednesday 26th September

Tonight I'm seeing Yacht Boy for dinner, followed by music. I'm looking forward to it as I haven't seen him for two weeks. A weekend work commitment got in the way of a second weekend's sailing and I'll be away again this weekend for a job interview abroad.

Even though I like both Fencing Boy and Yacht Boy, they're not quite snagging the raging attention junkie that lurks in me. They're both good-looking and great company. I want them physically and Fencing Boy is a top-notch lover, and passionate and jealous to boot. But there's still no real compulsion for me to be with either of them exclusively. After all, Fencing Boy will always text instead of ringing, or will just not call for two weeks. And Yacht Boy's lied to me about where he lived, was out of touch from May till August and doesn't always reply when texted.

Compare them to the Colonel who was an overweight, obnoxious, two-timing charmer who knew just how to give me the fixes of attention I craved, or KB who'd shower me with more tasteful affection, and drive me to the airport at the crack of dawn two days before Christmas even though I hadn't yet slept with him.

Wednesday 10th October

Went to the theatre with Tall Boy tonight.

My friend Pippa was in a new version of a Shakespeare play and my flatmate and another male friend came too. Tall Boy knows them from my birthday party and was his usual, sociable self.

Comfort, cosiness, familiarity. His finger stroking mine, my arm behind him, my hand in his. What *is* this?

I need to talk to him and have it out. We won't be working together much longer so who cares, really. I should let him know I love him and see what he plans to do about it. Probably nothing but he just feels so right to me that I can't help it. And I think I'm never going to get over him unless I bring it to a head.

'Shame I couldn't take you home tonight,' he texted me afterwards. He knows I'm such a sure thing and I hate myself for it. I can't stand the thought of lying next to him in bed and feeling the emptiness between us.

Tuesday 16th October

Fencing Boy dumped me via Facebook. Now that *is* class. After ignoring me all week, he emailed, 'I would like the friendship you are offering, but without the physical thing. Hope that's OK with you.' No, that's not OK with me. We'd last had sex while drinking in a posh hotel with friends. He pushed me up against a door frame in an upstairs corridor and banged away from behind. I came and he didn't. Fortunately the guest whose room it was didn't choose that moment to pop out of the door. After that there was another night when he slept over but was too grumpy and hung-over to even take me up on the offer of a shower, let alone a shag.

Still it would have been nice to know what went wrong. I guess I've got myself to blame for shagging him without considering the emotional fallout. He texted a little more to explain that he wants me in his life as a friend but he 'doesn't do fuck buddies'. My adoring glances into new babies' eyes during a walk in the park probably played another part in putting this relationship to sleep prematurely. Or maybe I shouldn't have taken him along when I went to meet an ex-flatmate's new baby daughter . . . He didn't even want to hold her. I suppose he's not comfortable with multi-dating, or dating broody women, which is his prerogative, but he could at least have slotted a coffee into his busy schedule to let his 'great friend' know in person, couldn't he?

At least Yacht Boy's managed to let me know why he hasn't been in touch. 'Work nightmares.' *I* should be having work nightmares. The clock is ticking and I still don't have a new job lined up.

Tuesday 23rd October

Why is it that when we break up with someone there's always a friend on hand to say, 'Make sure you're happy being single before you find new love.' To put this nifty piece of advice into a different context, would you tell someone who's just got the sack to make sure they're happy being unemployed before they got a new job? Or if someone loses a leg in an accident, should they be happy on one leg before they're rewarded with a pros-thetic? Or if you lose your friends should you try being Billy-no-mates before you find new buddies? Or stay lying on the ground when you fall off a horse?

If we realise that people aren't very happy being on the dole or on one leg, or having no friends and lying in the mud while their horse canters off, why do we assume that the new dumpee should be 'happy being single'?

People have jobs, legs, friends, mounting blocks and partners for a reason! I mean, sure, you can get by without them, but isn't life more fun and much easier if you have them?

I refuse to be 'happy being single' when I'd far rather share both the good and the bad of life with another person whom I truly love and who loves and appreciates me.

Thursday 25th October

Am having to negotiate and juggle two rival job offers – a good feeling to be in demand, but a bit unsettling that one company wants me to move abroad, and the £ sign in front of the amazing salary they offered initially, suddenly changed into a euro. I'd have to rent out my flat and put a lot of my things into storage, which seems a bit silly after moving in just a year ago. Ah well, takes my mind off juggling the boys.

Friday 26th October

Tired of sitting on a heap of loose ends I texted Yacht Boy to find out how I was supposed to interpret his silence this past month. He called immediately and apologised. Been very busy with work. I've been busy too, with work and life and men, but I still make time to send a text message or two. What potential is there in this relationship? If I decided to get involved with him in earnest, would I still be happy to wait a month for him to call back? Would it make him more reliable if I decided he could be the one I'd like to settle down with? Makes me glad I didn't seduce him on his boat.

Wednesday 31st October

'Waking up next to you only reminds me of what I don't have,' I told Tall Boy one morning last summer. And he just ruffled my hair and told me to stop having silly thoughts. After that I didn't let him sleep in my bed any more.

Thursday 1st November

A few weeks ago I spotted a poster of an adorable baby at my gym, with a phone number for the council adoption information line. I copied it down then dithered about calling for a few days, then finally rang up and found out about an information day.

I took a gay friend along with me as he was crashing on my sofa and didn't have a key, and because I needed the moral support – I'd cried on his shoulder about my broodiness and lack of decent men enough times. The other thing was, it was specifically for mixed-race couples aiming to adopt children from an ethnic minority, so with him I'd feel less self-conscious and would be able to concentrate on what was being said rather than feeling out of place as a single white person.

I wasn't sure what to expect. I just wanted to know what my options were if I hadn't met Mr Right by the time I am thirty-five. It was pretty enlightening, but it was also a lot of food for thought. For example it's rare to find babies looking for homes; usually it's slightly older kids who've grown up neglected, abused or who have lost a parent to drugs. It's not as though you get a cute little bundle which is a blank slate.

What if the child I was interested in had a bratty older brother or sister who came as part of the package? Was I grown-up enough to deal with that? Did it matter if it turned out that the child was physically or mentally disabled in some way? Would I have to consider which school they went to and where I lived if they didn't want to be separated from their friends? What kind of contact, if any, would I want with the birth parents? And what if I was blinded by appearances and my arms' longing to hold the 'perfect' child when I should be snaffling up some little runt who might have less of a chance?

And then, of course, there's the small matter of how suitable the adoption people think I am. You can adopt if you're single, but if you're in a couple you have to have been together for a minimum of two to three years to provide a stable background for the child. As a single, blonde and blue-eyed white female I was unlikely to qualify to take home a dark-skinned baby. It seemed ironic, given that there are scores of white single mums out there with brown babies who are genetically as white as they are black.

To underscore that irony, one of the speakers was a lady of West African heritage who had a daughter from a Caribbean background. The mother hadn't even been to the Caribbean, let alone to the specific island (I have, but there you go).

There are also all the technical difficulties of applying to adopt, getting financial assistance and arranging adoption leave. My head was swimming with considerations and notes for dealing with the bureaucratic procedure involved, but you have to remember it's all for the best interests of the children. My heart softened and my eyes welled up when I came across a magazine called 'Children who wait' which is a glossy catalogue of kids who want a 'for ever home' and a new family. I flicked through, eager to experience that 'instant connection' people often describe when seeing their future child for the first time.

It didn't happen – this time – but I left grateful that my friend had been there to keep me company, and wondering when was the best time to register my name with the agency. It might take eighteen months or more, so do I wait till the urge to have a child is uncomfortably strong or my finances are more settled? More unanswerable questions – but the experience filled me with hope that there's light at the end of the tunnel, man or no man.

12

Truth or Dare

WINTER 2007

Monday 5th November

I should love my new job because technically, as my flatmate pointed out today, 'You're just like that girl in *The Devil Wears Prada* – "a million girls would kill for her job, but she hates it".' Indeed.

The office is busy like a train station at rush hour, and contrary to what was promised in my interviews the tasks are tedious and people are constantly in my business. The little decisions I do get to make are frequently whipped out from under me at the last minute, rendering several days' work useless. Everyone wants me to find not one option when I book them a hotel but four or five, even though they'll only spend one night of their lives there. I asked the girl who is showing me the ropes whether this constant checking and double-checking of her work, followed by having to do it all over again, doesn't get frustrating. 'But this is what you get paid for,' she told me, and I bit my tongue rather than say I thought I got paid to use my brain, in case she took it as a dig at her. I've got to give her a break as she's only twenty-one and obviously dedicated to paying her dues so she can cut a swathe through the industry.

No wonder my predecessor left a nearly full plastic bottle of industrial-strength whisky in her bottom desk drawer. Judging by the state of the rest of it, she didn't use the alcohol for cleaning . . .

I have been drowning my sorrows in the company of my two dearest friends, Moët and Chandon.

Monday 12th November

Well, that didn't last long! I got the sack on Friday. That's what? A week? Good job I don't have a flat full of precious adopted kiddies. Not good for the old confidence, let me tell you, not good at all. *But* if you add up the bizarre hours, the way the job followed me home, the lack of communication from my bosses and total absence of responsibility for me, oh and the hopelessly inadequate computer system, you can see that this wasn't exactly the job for me. 'It's just not working out,' they told me, and I had to agree. And it's not going to work out for them unless they buck up their ideas, their computer network and their expectations.

Came home to my friend the sofa and decided to have a texting session. No response from the Sailor in Scotland, but Canada Boy phoned back for a nice long chat. He invited me to come and stay in Toronto, although maybe that will have to wait till I have a paying job. Then I texted French Doctor, to see if he was feeling mischievous.

'I am wearing my white coat and am hard for you, thinking of your ass and pussy,' he typed.

'Oh, a horny doctor,' I fired back, my mind working overtime and imagining him stroking himself under his scrubs, a stethoscope hanging round his shoulders.

'I can't wait to taste your pussy again, Sienna, so hot and sweet.'

'I imagine your tongue on my clit, fingers inside me . . .'

'I am in my room, thinking of you and playing . . . ' he continued as I began to get wet, then begged, 'Send me pictures.'

So I pulled down my sweat pants and knickers to reveal the soft, furry outline of my pussy. I've begun to grow my hair back from the narrow, summer landing strip and bare lips to a more womanly shape, trimmed but triangular, which I prefer.

'DON'T STOP BABY, SHOW ME MORE! SHOW ME YOUR PUSSY AND ASS . . . YOU DRIVE ME CRAZY! LOVE IT!' he texted in response.

This was a challenge. I mean, how does one take pictures of one's own butt? I began to empathise with a friend who once enlisted my help to take photos of her tits for her long-distance boyfriend. And it was midnight and there was no one to ask for help. Not that I know anyone who I can ask to take photos of my bare bum for another man.

I slipped my trousers down further, listening out for my flat-mate's key in the door (this would be a little hard to explain to her), reached my phone round and began snapping away.

First attempt: a peachy round shape with a crack down the middle. Could be anything. Not very appealing.

Second attempt: too close. Is it a loaf of bread? A flesh-coloured duvet?

Third: bingo! You can just about see the top of my legs and the edge of my pulled-down knickers, my cheeks at a saucy angle.

'My favourite ass in the world, so beautiful,' he gushed, 'and soon will be mine again. I am almost ready to come, baby, one more shot for me?'

I complied and he loved it: 'U are a girl for everything! Smart, interesting, beautiful, sexy, what a deadly combination! How can I resist? PS. Waiting for photo. Still hard.'

So that earned him a close-up crotch shot, just to shut him up – a bit graphic but you couldn't see my face. 'As you can see, I need a manicure,' I commented, referring to the chipped polish on the fingers holding my lips apart. 'Do I get to see a picture of your cock?' I asked, imagining him pulling aside his doctor's coat to reveal a huge erection, just before dashing off to A&E.

So let's hope this leads to a plane ticket and a well-deserved shag break on a smooth-sanded beach. And there you have it. While most people would trawl the web for vacancies and be running to the post box at midnight with a pile of CVs, I was kneeling on the sofa with my arse in the air, and my camera clicking away.

Maybe I need to take my career a bit more seriously?

Thursday 15th November

Today I received my fourth proposal of marriage. And this one was serious.

Not Yacht Boy. Not Fencing Boy throwing pebbles at my window at midnight, waving a bunch of flowers and begging for forgiveness. Not French Doctor, fresh from an easyJet flight and brandishing a ring bought in duty-free. Not a regretful KB nor Cashmere, nor the Pilot.

It was an unusual request for a first date, but I suppose we have at least known each other for years. And no, it's not Canada Boy. It's a new player, Country Boy. Let me recap.

We met when he was interviewing me for a job which I didn't get and at the time I didn't realise it, but he's actually three years younger than me. Like KB he has the physique, bespoke suits and confidence of a much older man. For some reason, even though he didn't give me the job, I seem to have made an impression, and cornered a little part of his mind. When I emailed all my old contacts to find out about job opportunities he latched on and has been oh-so-harmlessly 'stalking' me on the internet ever since, to my bewilderment.

It took me a while to catch up to the fact that he was trying earnestly to flirt with me in emails, and I didn't take his advances very seriously at all, deciding instead to put him off with the line, 'I want to meet a guy I can get married to and have children with,' which has, after all, worked like magic at getting rid of guys I both did and didn't want to get to know better in the past.

This seemed to bounce off Country Boy, and so I found myself sitting opposite him at a swanky bar this evening. Well, after I turned up late. A whole hour late. Embarrassing and out of character yes, but perhaps a subconscious effort to put him off my scent.

It didn't work. He ordered a bottle of wine I didn't request, paid for my food even though he wasn't hungry, and set about divulging family secrets, name-dropping left, right and centre and, well, proposing.

Unless a wannabe suitor follows through with a carat-laden gift, I've learned not to take proposals seriously, but it was still flattering. But. I don't fancy him. And he made the unfortunate mistake of telling me he 'used to date someone famous' who was 'now like a sister to him' (hello, Pinocchio and his ex!)

'Is her picture on your fridge?' I asked him, in case this was the norm with all men and their exes who are 'just like a sister'.

'No,' he replied, 'but yours would be.' And he proceeded to show me a couple of photos of him and her on his phone, wearing identical glasses. How cute.

I found myself wondering how his passion would translate to the bedroom, his slightly tubby hands on my flesh like KB's big paws, exposing and exploring my nipples in his club's library. Uninvited attention and a good mauling forced on me, yet not unwelcome or rejected . . . A warm tingle spread from my pussy up my spine.

If he thinks he really wants to marry me, let him prove it. Who am I to say I don't want to get to know him better while he spoils and flatters me, and waits patiently for an hour to have me listen to him for a while, and gets nothing in return save a peck on the cheek.

'A feast for my senses,' he texted me after I left in a hurry, needing to be at my Power Point class and being late, 'let's do it again soon.'

He wants me to come shooting one weekend and for 'another drink, a later, longer one', not to forget 'log fires and chestnuts, dressing for dinner, country church, mulled wine . . . and Sienna, can I just say you are beautiful far, far beyond words.'

Attention, flattery, a boy too young for me, a boy I don't fancy, posh, Cashmere, KB . . . My head tells me one thing, and yet my stupid heart disagrees, encouraged by my neglected pussy!

Monday 19th November

I did it. I took the plunge.

Last night Country Boy squired me to a bar for a Bellini, before we moved on to a party. Much flirting and flattery ensued, but every time I asked him why he wanted to marry me he just replied, 'Why not?'

'Are you sure you want kids this young?' I asked him, half teasing, half serious, my ever-increasing broodiness being the biggest driving force behind my desire to tie the knot. 'When was the last time you changed a nappy?'

'We'd have a maid for that,' he replied in all seriousness.

'You can afford a *maid*?' I asked him with an ironic smile. He nodded and I laughed out loud. Get him! 'An au pair, perhaps,' I conceded, 'but then I'd have to worry about you running off with her.'

'I don't think any man who has you would run off with the au pair,' he countered smoothly.

What I should have said was, 'I'm sorry, but I don't fancy you and I can't imagine promising to wake up next to you for the rest of my life,' but my body, fuelled by champagne and his undivided attention, seemed to think otherwise.

'Chelsea registry office, Westminster Abbey, a beach, me in a white suit – you'd look divine in white,' and other nuggets led us to sit down in a corner, and I noticed the wetness between my legs. My pussy was swimming, swollen and throbbing, for I-don't-know-what reason.

I sat facing a man three years my junior who was wearing a gold-buttoned, double-breasted blazer, glasses below his shiny forehead. I should have been running for the ladies' and checking the windows to find an escape route, not hanging on his every word. I giggled more at him than with him, but in the back of my mind his hands were sneaking between my legs on a four-poster bed in a dusty manor. My smiles and flirting spurred him on and made him bolder, until his fingers rested against my back on the crocheted shrug I had thrown over my corset.

'I am disappointed I can't feel your skin through this,' he commented. Half waiting for him to brush the shrug aside, I leaned into his touch and listened to him drone on about country weekends, shooting and my divine presence. I thought I'd be disappointed if he followed through on these promises, but if he did I'd be scandalised and unsure how to react. It all seemed like make-believe. I consulted my inner bullshit detector, that infallible device I used to frequently ignore in my teens and early twenties, but it didn't so much as squeak, so I can safely assume he meant every word, or at least, he did at that very moment.

I went home alone. He sent me a text saying, 'I could never grow tired of waking up next to you in a thousand years. And I wouldn't want you any less.' Wonderful words. I was wide awake at midnight.

So I sent a text to Tall Boy, offering myself up on a plate. And a short while later he pulled up in a taxi with a friend who was visiting, and swept me off to his 'castle' in the arse-end-of-nowhere, where they also have shootings, but pheasants aren't generally involved.

On the back seat he held my hand and looked at me in such an excited, charming way that I could see his eyes sparkle in the half light. I am sure I was gazing back like a love-struck puppy too, squirming in my damp knickers.

We pulled up and he paid the cabbie, and then he led me and his friend in through the kitchen with its sticky floor and piles of dirty dishes, to the living room which was decorated with calendars of girls in bikinis, stacks of old lads' mags, a pile of dusty coins on a shelf, beer cans full of cigarette ash and enough empty bottles to open a small recycling facility. I've seen younger sofas in skips. Mind you, a quick glance told me that I'd read or wanted to read almost every book there, and his clothes were clean and folded by the ironing board, and he seemed to find the state of the place as hilarious as I did.

There was only one thing for me to do: accept his offer of a generous (filthy) glass of Sauvignon Blanc, take my socks off to wriggle my toes to Iron Maiden and grab the inflatable guitar for an impromptu air-guitar riff while waiting for the booze to numb my sense of aesthetics enough to get back on my wave of passion.

How, I wondered, did I get from Bellinis in a fancy bar and visions of country house weekends to Straight Nightmare for a Gay Eye?

His mate disappeared upstairs to the spare room and we were finally alone. Tall Boy gathered me up in a big hug. 'I have missed you,' he whispered, and led me up to his bedroom. I had missed him too. I was struggling to remember when was the last time we'd slept together – some time in the summer I think, and then only sexless cinema and theatre trips after that.

'When we did it upstairs at your old office I came so fast because I was so excited. That was the hottest sex I have ever had,' he confided in a thick voice, his hands caressing my body.

When he envelopes me in his arms I feel totally wrapped up, at home, swept along by our passion. I really do forget the world around me, just like the cliché. His soft lips and hair, his probing tongue and his big, gentle hands could be part of my universe for ever.

'I can still remember the first time I saw you,' he said. 'Yes,' I replied, and kissed his neck, 'I was wearing a really short red dress.' 'I know,' he smiled, 'I thought – this girl won't like me – but you did.' 'Of course I do,' I kissed him on the lips, deeply. 'I've fancied you for over a year,' he went on, and it sounded like a mixture of stating the obvious and a candid confession. This much is clear, I thought, feeling his erection against me. He stripped all my clothes off and pushed me onto the bed.

'You are like my childhood sweetheart,' he said, right against my ear, 'I love your beautiful face, your hair, your soft skin. You are this beautiful, smart girl with a hot body ... ' and he sounded like he meant it. My bullshit detector was silent, or drowned out, but somewhere in me a small voice asked, if he feels like this, why doesn't he *want* me? Not just as a fuck buddy, a fun girl to hang out with or the ex-colleague he fancies – but a companion, a partner, a girlfriend, whatever you want to call it.

He went down on me for ages, his tongue busy probing me and flicking against my clit with just the right pressure, his fingers inside me, getting wet to the wrist. I moved one of his fingers into my ass and came hard, clutching him to me tightly as my body rocked on the waves of my orgasm. He pulled himself over me and plunged his hard cock into me, so deep it hurt. I wanted him desperately, pulling him into me, kissing and licking his neck as he thrust into me. He stopped to pull out a condom which I rolled onto him with my mouth, playing with his cock and balls till he pushed me away and plunged back into me.

His arms were wrapped right round my back, our legs were intertwined as we rocked and shuddered against each other, locked together. There was no mistaking when he came; I thought he would pass out. The way his cock expanded in me, spurting against me, him groaning and gasping with pleasure as he spasms again and again, pumping into me.

It was so intense that tears rolled down my face. He kissed my cheeks and eyes, the salt of the tears mixing with sweat. I rested my head on his chest as he pulled me close, stroking my hair, my back, my arm.

'I have a confession to make,' I said, softly, 'I am utterly in love with you.'

He murmured something incomprehensible, and I realised by the rising and falling of his chest that he was almost asleep. Lying there in his arms, exhausted, happy, the corner of my mouth still salty with tears and the room spinning from the alcohol, I knew he wasn't going to return my confession, if he'd even heard it. Minutes later, I was asleep too.

Wednesday 28th November

After my confession to Tall Boy the other night, all was suspiciously quiet between us. I was half proud of myself for being brave and coming clean, half hoping he hadn't seen my tears in the dark, and that he would blame my words of love on the alcohol and general atmosphere of our post-coital fug.

Today I tried to find out what night that office Christmas party was that he'd invited me to this week. 'There will be loadsa clients there,' he texted back, 'why don't we just meet up when I am back next week? Am away this weekend.' Oops, silly me: and I thought that the clients present would be the *point* in having a glammed-up, tall blonde on his arm?

I called him to give him a piece of my mind, which, of course, turned into mindless flirting and general catching up and being filled with happiness upon hearing his voice. His explanation left me feeling less fobbed off than his text had done, and I wished him a good night and a fun trip, vowing to myself that I would delete his number and never see him again this side of Christmas, for the sake of my own sanity. Then I rang Tall Boy back.

'You're very smooth.'

'I've been called a lot of things,' he joked, 'but never that.'

'Why not? How would you define smooth?'

'Someone who has a lot of lines, who tells people what they want to hear.'

'Well, you told me a lot of nice things that I wanted to hear very much, like saying your parents would love to meet me, or you'd fancied me for a year, or that I was your dream girl.'

'That is true.' Without seeing him I could hear the smile in his voice. 'But those weren't lines. My parents *would* love to meet you. My mum's always banging on at me to bring girls home.'

'I'm away next week,' he continued, 'but I'll give you a ring when I get back.'

'Actually,' I paused, 'I'm thinking the opposite.'

'What do you mean?' he asked in a confused voice.

'I think it might be best if you don't call. Every time we see each other we have a great time, but we're not just friends, are we? Friends don't hold hands and go on dates.'

'True.'

'You told me you don't want a girlfriend,' I went on, 'but you've given me mixed messages from the moment I clapped eyes on you, and I just want everything to be out in the open. It's hard for me to see you and feel really close to you and to hear all these things from you and then not see you again for ages. This isn't the kind of relationship I want. I want to be with someone who's there for me, who gets me a card for my birthday and just wants to be with me. And you want to get pissed with your mates, and have fun. And there's no reason why you shouldn't, but it hurts me that you see other people.'

'But so do you, Sienna,' he protested. For the first time I could detect something like jealousy or mild disapproval in his voice.

'Of course. But the difference is, it bothers me and it doesn't bother you.'

He stayed quiet.

'I'm not sure if you heard me the other night when I said I'm in love with you. I needed to let you know how I feel because you can't read my mind. You told me you thought I'd been busy since the summer, but I was just trying to hold back and protect myself from getting hurt by getting too close to someone who doesn't really want to be with me.'

I knew what was coming. If he'd wanted to be with me exclusively he would have put in the time, he'd have tried to be reliable, genuinely caring and consistent, and he would have stopped seeing other people and wanted me to do the same.

'I'm sorry,' he said, noticing how my voice had filled up with tears, 'maybe we should just be friends then. I'd like that.'

And that was that. The conversation ended without us knowing when we might see each other again, but it's probably for the best. I have enough friends already. The only thing I'm lacking is a man who wants to make the transition from lover to husband.

Epilogue

In a funny way I'm grateful to him. It felt good to have an open, honest conversation.

He'd said it himself: he'd fancied me for a year, which is great, but he also decided that this wouldn't mean the beginning of a loving relationship and I need to accept this.

I knew he didn't want a girlfriend, so I kept my options open and yet I developed feelings for him. It's time to admit my own responsibility in this: I decided to get my romantic hopes up despite my gut feelings.

I couldn't stop myself saying 'I love you' but it felt like something much bigger, like an admission that I was finally able to love someone again, and I could say it out loud and fuck the consequences! Talking to him has made me realise that I am no longer afraid to fall for someone and get hurt, and I don't worry any more that I will risk anything by telling the person I love about it. After sharing my expectations with him I feel much closer to myself and my own hopes and desires.

So, he's not perfect. Show me someone who is. I'm glad I can love and accept him for who he is, but I cannot force him to love me back. And I am *really* glad I don't have to be the one to tidy up his crusty house.

It didn't kill me to say the words out loud, and it won't kill me to walk away from him, now that I know he doesn't want the same as me. Because I was honest with him he won't be able to 'have' me any more in a way I've now realised I don't want because it feels more like a compromise than freedom. Because he was honest with me I don't feel compelled to rip up his bikini calendars or stick fish under his floorboards in misguided revenge. Not all men lie, like Pinocchio – I actually feel sorry for *him* now because he was in love with an ex who didn't want him any more and instead tried to make do with little old me. If I don't want to end up like him, it's up to me to recognise who is right for me and who isn't, and I think my experience with the men I met over the last few years should really help me with this.

I'll aim to keep clear of someone who is focusing all his attention and money on the pursuit of his career, like the Pilot, or someone who needs to grow up a bit more before taking on responsibilities, like Sweet Ex and KB, or someone who talks about love but doesn't know how to show it – like Cashmere. I don't want to be taken in by someone who has all the expensive toys but doesn't share my sense of humour, like Rugby, or someone who has an exotic hobby but no time, like Yacht Boy, or who has the amazing body but limited communication skills (BBP). I refuse to put up with disrespect like I got from the Colonel, I want to be honest about what I'm looking for and not play games like Dance Boy, and above all I don't want to end up like Samantha with a gorgeous baby but no daddy for support because I didn't take my time.

The discovery that bedding multiple suitors is more about ego than true love doesn't mean I regret my experiments in dating, but I now want something more substantial.

I was open-minded about the way my lovers wanted our relationships to play out in the past – booty calls, weekends away, soulmates who never see each other – but from now on I want to make a few conditions for men who date me.

It seems to me that my confession wasn't really for Tall Boy. It was more about saying the words out loud than about him hearing or reacting. A declaration of intent. I'm suddenly a lot clearer about what I really, truly want, and it's not Tall Boy, or KB, or the Pilot or a mindless fuck, it's someone who's in love with me, and a relationship where that love is enough for both of us.

Since Tall Boy helped me realise what I'm missing, I am optimistic that a perfect match for me and all my imperfections is still out there somewhere. I'm sure it'll be easier to recognise it when I find it.

'He's already born,' said my grandma in Holland.

At least, I should hope so.

Acknowledgements

For a number of years I had wanted to write an honest account of the men I'd met, slept with, dreamt of and fantasised about, but I didn't get started properly until I began my blog in August 2005.

For this, I would like to thank and credit the following people: Thea Newcomb, for setting up and maintaining www.soyouvebeendumped.com which has helped so many people after relationship breakdowns, and which provided me with a much-needed outlet for my early ramblings and a host of supportive dumpers and dumpees who could relate to what I was going through. Although I often chose to ignore Thea's advice about dating too soon (as you will have seen from this book), I am grateful I had SYBD to vent and turn to for support. Posting on the forum proved so therapeutic that I decided to start to record my new dating philosophy and all its triumphs and pitfalls in the blog which served as the blueprint to the book you are now reading. Thank you, Thea, for being an inspiration to the broken-hearted and for teaching me to make lemonade out of the lemons I was handed in life.

My wonderful mum, who never seems to grow tired listening to my dramas, and who suggested I join my first dating website. Thank you for being my rock, and never judging me.

My fantastic agent, James Wills, for his patience and advice, right from the first time we met when this book was still just a speck on the horizon, through to the present day. Thank you for your help in every stage of this book, for your professionalism and integrity.

Charlotte Cole at Ebury, thank you for all your comments and input, and Rachel for remembering my email.

P.L., thank you for letting me look after Z, whose love meant so much to me in a difficult time and who was a willing recipient for my need to mother someone, whose laughter brightens up a dull day, and whose tears could never stain it.

My sister, for being honest, fierce and 'normal', and to H.L. for being like a sister when I needed one close by.

My lovely blog friends, whose comments have been a great support over the years, thank you for sharing, for bearing with me and for your genuine warmth.

All the men I have met in my life, mentioned or not – thank you for the laughs, the snogs, the dinners, the cocktails, the drives, the conversations, the flights, the massages, the parties, the dances, the orgasms, the tears, the emails, the sailing trips, the experiences without which this book would be very dull indeed. Thank you for showing me which qualities are important to me in a partner.

The professionals whose help I received during dark times – writing might be great therapy, but it wasn't the only assistance I had with dragging myself out of a period of depression. Thanks to my counsellors, the GP who referred me to group therapy, the rather detached doctor who led these sessions (you don't have to love them for this to work), and the assortment of fellow patients (never underestimate the humour in a group entitled 'Overcoming Depression'), I managed to escape the hole I'd slipped into and reclaim my sunny personality. I would urge anyone who finds they no longer recognise themselves to seek professional help and return to a mental state where they can love themselves again.

I would also like to thank the doctors and medical staff who treated me (with dignity, humour, creams and cryo) during my embarrassing HPV outbreak and who reassured me about how common it is. May this book help fellow sufferers to know they aren't alone, and urge the mothers of pre-pubescents to get them vaccinated.

A.F., thank you for being a loyal friend, and for taking me to a comedy club when I most needed it. Your girlfriend is a lucky lady.

A.J., thank you for your angelic assistance and healing.

D.L., for you, part of me sometimes considers converting to Judaism. May you always have love, polyamorous or not.

S.F., thank you for the personal training sessions, and for guiding me through the maze with wit and humour.

I am donating a percentage of my proceeds from this book to the *Guardian*'s Katine appeal in Uganda, which supports AMREF to help local women:

'In addition to providing better quality classrooms, latrines and washrooms, AMREF has now influenced the local government to draft female teachers into the community primary schools who act as positive role models for girls and give pastoral support. Empowering women in the community is key to effective long term attitudinal change in Katine.' (Craig Pollard, Amref UK)